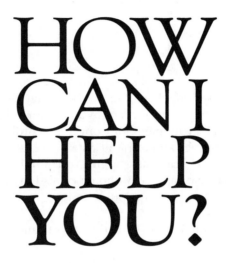

HOW CAN I HELP YOU?

THE MOST IMPORTANT QUESTION
IN BUSINESS AND IN LIFE

by

M. Walter Levine

with Virginia Juliano

How Can I Help You?
The Most Important Question in Business and In Life.

© 2010 M. Walter Levine

Printed in the United States of America.

First Edition

ISBN: 978-0-578-06867-1

MWL Enterprises
P.O. 355
Greens Farms , CT 06838

Cover photo by
Robert Mitchell
www.mitchellphotos.com

Cover and book design
Suzanne Annunziato   Printing: Signature Book Printing

DEDICATION

This book is dedicated to Fritzie,
without whose love and support
I would never have been able to
"TURN THE PAGE."

"It is what it is."

— M. Walter Levine

To my sweetheart, Chuck,
who always dares me to
dream bigger.

— Virginia Juliano

TABLE OF CONTENTS

FOREWORD
By Virginia Juliano

"The power to question is the basis of all human progress."
— Indira Gandhi

When I met Marvin "Walter" Levine for lunch one August afternoon in Westport, CT. I was not expecting my life to change. But it did. That's the effect that Walter tends to have on people. My husband Charles (or Chuck, as I call him) and I anxiously walked into Walter's office, a comfortably outfitted greenhouse at the edge of a beautiful waterfront property. His long time assistant sat at a desk across the room from his. His desk was scattered with yellow-orange buck-slips, post-its, photos, trophies, plaques, certificates, you name it. It was a bit of a mess, but an organized mess.

A few weeks prior, Chuck had mentioned to a friend how upset he was about a high school chum's 12 year old daughter who had brain cancer and was basically wasting away because of an inability to keep down any food due to her treatment. Without a moment's hesitation his friend recommended that my husband contact Walter Levine. "This guy knows everyone, and I mean everyone, in the medical field, who has anything to do with cancer. You have to talk to him." So Chuck gave him a call. Walter was very friendly, and open to chatting, but when Chuck explained the situation. Walter's tone turned very serious. He asked a list of questions regarding the girl's age, her condition, her treatment to date. He told Chuck that he would make a few calls and get back to him.

An hour later, Walter called back. "Do you have a pen?" he asked. He gave Chuck the name and number of a doctor who specialized in the type of cancer our friend's daughter had. He said that the doctor was expecting their call, and they would be able to get an appointment within a week, even though the wait list for this doctor was normally months long. Chuck thanked Walter, but before they hung up they talked a bit more, and Walter discovered that we had a home in nearby Rowayton, CT. Walter was ecstatic. "You must come for lunch! Bring your wife! I would love to meet you both!" he exclaimed. So that's how I wound up in the greenhouse on that fateful day. I walked in not knowing what to expect and not especially happy to be using up one of my scarce vacation days to have lunch with a man I'd never met, and not lounging on the beach, where I wanted to be. We drove up to an unassuming entrance on Westport's Beachside Avenue, the toniest of tony locations in this very wealthy beachside community. We stopped at the electronic gates, pressed the button and announced ourselves. The gates swung open. "Not too shabby," I said to my husband. We drove through the gates and past the garage that could've housed at least 20 cars, where we were told to park. Beyond the garage was the main house, a large brick structure, and beyond that we saw a vast expanse of the beautiful Long Island Sound.

We parked in front of the garage and walked up the path to the greenhouse office. As we did, the door swung open and we were greeted by an ebullient and impeccably dressed man of about 60. He had a full head of perfectly coiffed grey hair, a rosy glow and a smile that lit up his handsome face. "Charles! Virginia! I'm so happy you're here. Welcome." Walter gave us a big, warm hug hello and indeed made us feel completely welcome. He had tuna sandwiches and diet coke with potato chips waiting for us. We'd brought an apple ring from a local Norwalk bakery for dessert. Walter said that it looked amazing and he told his assistant to remind him to stop by the bakery next time he went to Norwalk to visit his son.

And so it began. We ate our tuna sandwiches as we chatted. Walter told us one story after another about this business that he owned, and that business that he started, and another business that he sold. I couldn't really follow. He also showed us tons of pictures of him with various celebrities, even Mother Theresa. Then he showed us a picture of him in a hospital bed. He looked about 90 years old, weighed about 90 lbs and had no hair. I couldn't believe it was the same guy, and I couldn't believe that the 90 lb man in the photo made it through alive, never mind the picture of energy and health that stood before me.

We chatted through lunch about many things, including mutual acquaintances. Coincidentally, Chuck's childhood baseball coach was a friend of Walter's. When I casually mentioned that I grew up in Brooklyn, Walter practically jumped out of his chair. "You did??!! Me too!!! I knew I liked you," he smiled. He told more stories about more businesses and even more people that he knew. Still having some trouble following the thread, I asked him what he did for a living and he practically exclaimed, "Everything!" Hmmm. Interesting.

We also talked about the book that Chuck was finishing — his second. When Chuck noted that I had basically served as editor for his first book, Walter looked me straight in the eye and said in a very serious tone, "I want you to help me write my book." I smiled, not thinking he was serious. "I'm not kidding," he continued. "I like you and I know that you can help me. I have lots of stuff written down on paper, but I don't know what to do with it. You can turn it into something. I know you can. And we're both from Brooklyn. Come on, it's destiny."

When you speak to Walter, you get the feeling that anything is possible. He's infectious. I have never met anyone with such unbridled enthusiasm. And he has absolutely no qualms about expressing it — fully. I must admit, that day I didn't really believe that he was serious about me writing his book. But after a slew of calls and emails throughout the following weeks, as well as a shipment of his hand-written notebooks, I began to take him seriously. That's how Walter is when he has his mind set on something — relentless. So we put together an action plan to get the notes into a digital format, so that I could begin editing, then I created the outline and concept for this book.

Walter's life has undoubtedly been varied and interesting. Although how he got to where he is from where he came from is a great story, it was his continued triumph over multiple and severe setbacks and the absolute belief that he could do whatever he put his mind to that really interested me. As a devout reader of self-help books and an unofficial student of psychology, I was fascinated by his attitude, but the fact that it was so foreign from what I was used to, probably made it even more intriguing to me. I'd say that I was raised with more of a focus on limiting potential hurt and disappointment rather than reaching for the stars. Trying to balance a desire for growth and accomplishment with the pull to stay within the accepted norms my Italian-American background has sometimes been a struggle for me. So something about this man and his unapologetic zest for life and his "anything is possible" outlook was hard to resist. It was almost like catnip to me. I felt a deep need to dissect it and find out more.

Walter doesn't drink or dabble in any mood altering substances. Never has. He is truly and unabashedly high on life. I'll be honest, sometimes I just don't get it. I don't get how someone can get up every day and have that much energy, passion, drive and hope. Especially after all that he's gone through. Although Walter is human, and thus has his foibles, the fact of the matter is, I've learned a lot from him and have tried to become more like him in many ways. I do believe that I met him for a reason. Maybe he's been put in my path on the way to my own personal journey towards growth, and since I've met him, I think I have changed – at least a bit.

It's taken an enormous amount of effort to try to break through that cynical, pessimistic shell that I'd been so proud of for so long. While writing this book, I've often asked myself, "How did he NOT give up? Would I have been able to do the same? Would I be able to do the same, even now?" I don't know for sure, but I certainly hope that at least some of his chutzpah has rubbed off on me. I guess it was very Walter-like for me to not only recognize the opportunity of his friendship when it presented itself, but to stick with it and with this book, even when I really, really wanted to give up. Walter's inspiration comes from his family and his religion, but most of all, himself. And although his parents came from humble beginnings, they never questioned his drive to succeed. They never tried to keep him "in his place" where "people like us" belong. As Walter has said, inspiration is in the doing, not in the thinking. I try every day to make hope, determination, resilience, relentlessness, adaption and flexibility my default state of mind, with varying degrees of success.

Since Walter and I started the process of writing this book quite a few years ago, both of our lives have gone through quite a lot of change and we've had to make many revisions and additions to the original draft, but we finally did it. We're finally here, and I believe we have something important to share. Walter's dedication to helping others, his unrelenting attitude of hope and the way he puts it into practice is, to me, a story of inspiration and a lesson on how to live life both personally and professionally. His question of *"How Can I Help You?"* is at the core of everything he does and its concept is both profound and simple at the same time. It's a twist on the golden rule perhaps, but Walter puts it into practice in his own unique way and his life story gives it a distinctive and colorful backdrop. I hope you'll agree.

INTRODUCTION
By M. Walter Levine

*"Hope is the companion of power and the mother of success;
for who so hopes strongly has with him the gift of miracles."*
– Samuel Smiles

Have you ever been given news that brought you to your knees? Has life ever thrown you a curve ball that took your breath away? Has your world ever been shaken with information that put a wobble in the course of your life? Would you like to have the power to control your destiny? Every once in a while you need a check up from the neck up. It helps to align your thinking to keep you on track so that your goals and mission are going in the same direction. Nobody ever said life was easy. Well, I wrote this book because I have surely been there. So, as we walk together through my journey, my wish is that you will find Hope and that it will carry you forward to the realization of your dreams. Live your life the way you want it to be. You need to know that what happens in your life is in your control. It is your choice.

You never know how and from where you will get guidance in life, and it my greatest hope and sincerest wish for you to take some of what I've learned and apply it to yourself and your personal journey — whether it's a fight against cancer, a fight against being poor, or whatever. When you add my principles to your every day choices, I guarantee that you will find the way less bumpy and more positive for your future. I will share my principles and the lessons I've learned during my journey from going from "Nuttin' to Something" (more on that later) by asking the simple question, "How Can I Help You?"

In 1991 my doctors informed me that over 90% of my body had cancer. They had essentially thrown in the towel as far as my treatment was concerned. I wasn't given much hope. That was nineteen years ago. What did I do? Well, I fought through the fear, got angry, got excited, consulted with others, visualized and prayed. This book is for all of you who thought of giving up. My message to you is: Please don't do it.

You can visualize a goal and you CAN make it happen — or at least give it your best try. And now you too will learn how.

Throughout this book, I share the hard-earned life lessons I've learned during my journey and illustrate how certain events and experiences in my life led me to these insights. They are as follows:

Life Lesson #1:   **Who Ever Said Life Was Easy?**

Life Lesson #2:   **There Are No Shortcuts**

Life Lesson #3:   **To Be Enthusiastic, You Gotta Act Enthusiastic**

Life Lesson #4:   **If You Do Nothing, You Get Nothing**

Life Lesson #5:   **How High Do You Want to Go? It's Up to You**

Life Lesson #6:   **When Opportunity Knocks, Answer the Door**

Life Lesson #7:   **Nothing is More Constant Than Change**

Life Lesson #8:   **Life Really is Beautiful; People Can Be Great When Given the Opportunity**

Life Lesson #9:   **It's Not Magic, Just Work Harder Than Everyone Else if You Want to Succeed**

Life Lesson #10: **You Can't Win if You Don't Play**

Life Lesson #11: **God Helps Those Who Help Others**

Life Lesson #12: **There is Always More to Learn**

As you read my story, I hope that despite the different circumstances of our lives, you will be able to identify with my struggle to overcome the many obstacles I've encountered and take away some helpful tools for your own personal journey. I suggest that you consider jotting down thoughts as they come to you, such as: How does this fit with my situation? How do I see my life right now? What steps can I take to reach my goal? How can I improve my circumstances?

I've done well for myself in the business world — I'm good at sales, and have literally come back from financial ruin multiple times using positive thinking, visualization and perseverance to achieve success. Upon reflection, I now see that I approached my cancer in many ways the same way I do business, but surviving cancer made me wish I could teach so many in the medical field to sell HOPE. A large number of them could learn a little more about how necessary hope is to a patient. Here's to the good guys, the medical professionals who care, truly care about their patients — you know who you are.

When I felt that I had finally "won the battle," the need to help others was enormous. I shared my knowledge and gave of myself, and let me tell you, the feeling is like no other. I am on top of the world when I am helping someone. I strongly believe that by helping others you are helping yourself. It would be my privilege for you to consider me your new friend who has survived the storm and now stands above the horizon, showing you where to look. Fight for your best life, never give up on what you want out of it, and please, whatever you do, do not listen to the nay-sayers. No one is immune from difficulties and nothing is more constant than change. But keep your sunny side up and know that you may (will) run into brick walls, conflict, self-doubt and bad days along the road. But you and your mind can conquer anything it believes it can.

Consider the classic children's book, The Little Engine That Could. Read it and believe it with all your heart — be that little engine. I think you can, and you can too. Listen to what successful people say, watch what they do, ask them questions about how things work. Watch and learn. Stay on top of your game. Cherish family. Build wonderful friendships, and think of these relationships as family. And when it happens enjoy the feeling. Surround yourself with supportive people, including your healthcare providers and healing professionals. And as Winston Churchill said, "Never, never, never, never give up." "Hope" is your visualization. Dream of success both in business and life, and love everything you do. I say: "Life is what you make it. So make it **great!**"

Part One

CHAPTER ONE
The Diagnosis

LIFE LESSON #1...
WHO EVER SAID LIFE WAS EASY?

"God gives nothing to those who keep their arms crossed."
— West African proverb

January 1991 - New York City

I had to wait three weeks for an appointment with Dr. Ron MacKenzie, one of the best diagnostic internists in the country. We were finally here in his waiting room at the Hospital for Special Surgery. However, looking back, the downhill slide had actually begun about a year before. It was the beginning of 1990, and the Taj Mahal Casino in Atlantic City had just opened. I love to gamble, so a group of friends and I took a trip to "christen" the new casino on its opening day. Dice in hand at the craps table, my nose started to bleed — not just bleed, gush — all over the beautiful new green felt table — quite a scene. The management hurried me into the first aid room and summoned the casino doctor. He immediately cauterized my nose, and that was that I went on my way. The craps table had to be closed down for the day for cleaning, but I was back at another one in no time, back to throwing the dice.

That day turned out to be the beginning of a regular occurrence of nosebleeds. Each time, I would go to the doctor's at Manhattan Eye, Ear, Nose and Throat Hospital, where they would cauterize and promptly send me home. Later that year, I started losing the hearing in my left ear, so I went to an ear specialist. The doctor performed a procedure that involved inserting a tube into my ear, which worked temporarily. Soon after that, though, I sneezed and broke three of my ribs. The only thing the doctors could do was tape and wrap me up.

I didn't put all of this together, and unfortunately neither did any of the doctors. I didn't have a General Practitioner at the time, as I had always been healthy. One of my best friends, Dr. Ralph Berardi, an OB/GYN who had delivered all my grandchildren, did regular check-ups on me. I did what I'd always done in my life, no matter the situation: I found the best doctor I could, and I got it taken care of as needed. It had always worked — up until now.

The pain in my back was so bad that I could hardly walk anymore. Ever since I took a fall on the tennis court back in October, the pain was constant and getting too intense to ignore. I'd first gone to see a sports medicine physician, the man who took care of the New York Giants football team. When he wasn't satisfied with the results of the X-rays and thought there was something more to the pain, he referred me to Dr. MacKenzie.

I had another fall the morning before the appointment. I was taking a shower and suddenly blacked out, falling so hard that my wife, Fritzie, heard the thud from the other room. When she ran in and saw me lying there, she tried to get me up but couldn't do it alone. She called downstairs for Willie, my houseman and driver. With their help, I was able to get up and onto the bed. They got me dressed, but I could hardly stand up. It was so unlike me. I'm usually strong, steady and full of energy. I thought that something had to be very wrong — and boy, was I right.

The drive into the city from Westport seemed like an eternity. Now here I was sitting in his office trying to get some answers. I could hardly sit I was in so much pain. More pain than I could have ever even thought possible. I could feel the other people in the packed office watching and feeling sorry for me, as I whimpered and cried uncontrollably. Although I could tell she was trying to be strong for me, my wife's face betrayed the absolute fear she felt in response to seeing her normally strong and energetic husband in this state. Seeing her eyes fill with tears every time she looked at me, as if she were saying with her eyes, "I wish I could take his pain away and give it to me," made me hurt even more. The door finally swung open and the nurse called out my name. The pain was beyond control, and I could not get up by myself, so the nurse called Dr. McKenzie to help. He quickly appeared in the doorway and they were able to get me in a wheelchair and into the examination room as everyone in the office looked on in sympathy and disbelief.

After the examination and many tests, Dr. Mackenzie calmly told me I'd have to stay overnight. I let go and let him take over. This decision was a difficult thing for a man like me to do, but I had no choice — I was in that much pain. They admitted me into the hospital, and when I woke up the next morning, I discovered that I had contracted a case of pneumonia (something I found out later was a somewhat common occurrence during hospital stays, especially in my very weak state.) It turned out that this condition was just the beginning of my adventure. My wife and children were in my room holding hands when one of the doctors they had turned me over to, came in and said the words that I will never forget: "You have cancer and it is very serious. Do you have your affairs in order?"

We sat there stunned. Although we didn't know the full extent of the diagnosis yet, he explained that it didn't look very good for me. I realized that I might have only a few days to live. "Wow," I thought. "This is some ending for a 53-year old, tough, hard-working Brooklyn guy who just reached a major goal in his life. Peace."

I was immediately transferred to New York Hospital for a battery of further tests — weeks of them. In fact, the doctors needed to stabilize the pneumonia first, so I was there for a month before they were able to even begin to think about treating me for the cancer. It was touch and go, and they had me on so much morphine that I have almost no memory of that time (looking back, it was probably a good thing). One thing I do remember was refusing to be in one of those small depressing hospital rooms I had been placed in which felt like a closet. I asked to pay the difference in price for a private room. The cost was $2000 per day, and it didn't matter to me at all. Money didn't have any value anymore. It was now comfort, views and surroundings. After years of struggle and hard work, I had the means to do this, so why shouldn't I?

They gave me the Harry Helmsley Suite that had a great view, three couches, several recliners and a private bath. A very long way from Brooklyn, I recall thinking at the time. I was in New York Hospital for 54 long days and longer nights while they tried to figure out exactly what we were up against. My family eased the discomfort and fear by keeping me busy and just being there. I had been blessed with so many flowers after the word spread that we gave most away to other patients in the children's ward. My beautiful hospital room and hallway smelled like a flower shop with over 300 arrangements and plants.

From my window, the view of the 59th Street Bridge and the East River gave life and movement to the fabulous city I loved so much. This was a renowned hospital in the heart of Manhattan, the greatest city in the world, in my opinion. I figured that if they knew anything about cutting edge cancer treatments and programs, it would definitely be here in my beloved New York with the best physicians. I trusted them to take over and heal me, to make me whole again. I had plenty of time to do nothing but get well, but I still had a lot to learn about the healthcare industry. After countless blood tests, X-rays and many other tests, the doctors informed us that the results were in and I had multiple myeloma, a type of cancer of the blood that specifically affects the plasma cells and bone marrow. The plasma cells, I soon learned were a very important part of one's immune system that produces antibodies to fight infection and disease. This was very serious. I was told my cancer was incurable. "Why now, God?," I cried.

One morning soon after, I awoke to find my team of lawyers and accountants and friends standing over my bed. It felt surreal, and I vividly recall asking, "What are you all doing here?" They had such serious looks on their faces, and they asked if I could think of anything else that needed to be taken care of regarding my estate. Did I want to give anything to anyone or make any additions or changes to my will? I promptly told them all to go straight to hell or at least back to their respective homes and offices. I had no intention of dying, and I planned to beat this thing called cancer. As far as I was concerned, the fight was on.

After almost a year of treatments and upwards of $440,000 in medical bills, I confronted the oncologist I'd been seeing, (I'll call him Dr. T). "I tried," he said, "but it doesn't look good." Then he told me that over 90% of my body was cancerous. "I know you're disappointed, but I've read all the books on your type of cancer, and I'm afraid there's nothing more we can do." At that moment, my fight for life got even stronger, and I shouted angrily, "You read the books on my cancer!?!? Well I want the guys who wrote the books on multiple myeloma!" Then I looked him in the eye and very slowly and firmly said, "Listen, I'm going to ask every person I know to help me hunt down the right doctor and the right treatment for me. I hope to God there's someone out there who can help me, and if I find out that there is someone somewhere who could've made a difference and you're not telling me, you can bet that I will come back here and take you with me." Without missing a beat, the doctor picked up the phone and arranged an appointment for me in Little Rock, Arkansas, with a top doctor originally from Germany by the name of Dr. Bart Barlogie at the Arkansas Cancer Research Center, the best of the best. The rest, as they say, is history. Well…almost.

■ Life Lesson 1: Who Ever Said Life Was Easy?

There is no guarantee that life is going to be smooth sailing, but that is no reason for you to just sit back and let life just happen to you. I share this story because when I was faced with the biggest fight of my life — which happened to be the fight **FOR** my life — I found myself having to reach back to my own history to tap into a fighting spirit and faith that I didn't even know I had in order to get me through. And I truly believe deep in my heart and soul that you can do the same.

During my stay in the hospital I had a lot of time to think about where and how I would get the mental and physical strength I would need to beat the odds. As I lay there in my hospital bed with I don't know how many needles stuck into me in the name of life, I had no idea if the drugs they were pumping into my veins were helping me or destroying my insides. Although the pain wouldn't let up, I tried not to lose myself in the morphine haze that was taking me out of myself and into a dream state. But I believed that I needed to stay in reality to survive, even though it was no picnic being there. In spite of the morphine, or maybe because of it, I began to have moments of clarity and flashes of childhood memories that reminded me just how tough I really was and always had been. I also realized that if I ever wanted to get out of that hospital I would need to be even tougher. I knew that the fight was on.

CHAPTER TWO
A Kid From Brooklyn

LIFE LESSON #2...
THERE ARE NO SHORTCUTS

"With money in your pocket, you are wise and you are handsome and you sing well too."
– Yiddish Proverb

*W*hile growing up, the one thing I knew for certain was that I had a very loving and giving family. My father, Harry Levine, was a Russian immigrant who left his homeland as a teenager. The story goes like this: In 1927, one fateful day in a town near Kiev, my grandfather, my father (who was fifteen at the time) and my Aunt Ida (thirteen) were walking down the street and stumbled upon a dead man in the gutter. My grandfather, Shia Gershonowitz, was a rabbi and carpenter whose wife (my grandmother) had just recently passed away from tuberculosis.

According to my father, in the dead man's jacket were three tickets for a steamer to Canada. They decided to act quickly and take advantage of their "luck." With nothing holding them back and no good reason not to, they headed straight to the dock, with only the clothes on their backs. Using the dead man's papers and name, the three boarded a steamer bound for North America. The dead man's name was Sam Levine, the name my grandfather decided to use for his new life.

People have said that things must've been pretty bleak for them to decide that this was the best option available to them. But I like to think that my grandfather's drive for something better and the ability to take advantage of an opportunity must have been incredibly strong and outweighed his fear of the risks involved. When the ship docked in Canada, they made their way to Toronto for a while and then headed south to New York's Lower East Side, finally settling in Borough Park, Brooklyn.

Mini-Lesson: *I think that this is an incredible example of courage. Imagine starting a whole new life with no money, no clothes – nothing. This always made me believe that even without a penny, you still have your name and your reputation, and that in itself is worth a lot. I think that knowing this about my family history gave me the courage to take chances, because I knew on a certain level that*

even if I lost everything (which I have done several times)
having my name, reputation and intellect is all one really
needs in this life to start over.

My grandfather soon remarried and at sixteen, my dad needed to help with the family finances. So Harry got a job at Star Corrugated Box Company in Maspeth, Queens, working the night shift, as it paid $18 more a month than the day shift. Still, there was no extra money for treats or movies or luxuries. As it turns out, my dad wound up working for the Etra Family, making cardboard boxes at Star for forty-seven years. He was well respected, loved and admired, as I would find out years later at his funeral. He always said that his co-workers were like a second family to him.

Mini-Lesson: *This is part of the "3 Family System" that I've come to believe in. Your first family is of course the one you are born into. Then, there is your family of friends. This is the family you choose for yourself. And then last but not least my father helped me to see that people you work with are your "working" family. This is the family you see every day and actually spend the most time with. Each "Family" sees a different side of you and gets to know you like no other.*

My mom, Faye Butler Levine, was one tough lady. She was born in Boston to Russian immigrants Sara and David Botlinksy (shortened to Butler when they came to America). "Pop" and "Bub" (my nicknames for my grandparents) lived with us in East Flatbush, Brooklyn until I turned fourteen. During my childhood, I remember my mom always having several jobs. In my early years, she worked in a lollipop factory during the daytime, putting sticks in the candy while it was warm. At night, she worked with our next-door neighbor, Claire Gutterman, selling Stanley Home Products, both door to door and through the many friendships she made. Claire's son, Joel Gutterman, and I are still close family to this day. Joely, or 1A, as I like to call him (he calls me 1B, since those were our apartment numbers), owns a CPA practice, and he's a great success, working hard just like his mom did.

Although my parents tried very hard to make a buck and gain a degree of success, they didn't make a lot of money. They never once stopped working very hard, though — and more importantly, they never stopped doing good deeds for people, each and every day. Every cent that my folks made was used to help family: my brother and I and my grandparents. We lived in a building on Rockaway Parkway in Brooklyn. At the time, I thought it was a pretty nice neighborhood. The buildings were cramped together, attached on both sides with a small slab of cement as a backyard. They were your basic tenements consisting of 72 families in each apartment building, with "Tar Beach" for city rooftop sunbathing. You just had to be sure to bring an old sheet with you or you would turn black from the warm tar.

One day, I asked my mom and dad for ten cents to go to the movies with my friends, Joely Gutterman and Alan Schwartz. Dad told me that if I wanted money, I had to earn it. Well, considering it was 1943, and there was a war going on, there weren't many job opportunities available to a six year-old kid. Even then, I must have realized on some level that because of my parents' circumstances, there was only so much that they could do for me. It seemed perfectly natural for me to take matters into my own hands and start my first business, although at the time I didn't realize it was a business. I just thought it was a way to make a few quick pennies to pay for a ticket to the movies. In retrospect, I realize that's exactly what it was — providing a service to others which I could do better, or make it easier for them than if they were to do it on their own. It also taught me that if you need anything, you have to work for it yourself. I think this was the beginning of my lifelong credo for business and life: "How Can I Help You?," which is basically finding out what people need and helping them get it.

So, with the little I had available to me, I looked around my neighborhood for ideas. I decided to take advantage of the resources that others left (or dropped) behind. I would go to all of the backyards of the crowded, six-story apartment buildings in my neighborhood, with my father's size 12 shoe box in tow, and pick up all the fallen clothespins. I took them home, washed them in the bathtub and dried them with a towel. Then I took my mother's red nail polish and put a small spot on the top of each so people would know that they were mine. Now that's branding! I proceeded to go around knocking on doors and selling them three for a penny. No one owned a washing machine or dryer in those days; women used a washboard in the kitchen sink to do laundry. They hung the clothes on clotheslines from the window to poles in the back of the buildings. The ladies appreciated my service, and before I knew it, they were knocking on my door placing their orders. They would give my grandmother money wrapped in pieces of newspaper and write down how many clothespins they needed and their address and apartment number for delivery.

From then on, I always had money in my pocket for my friends and I to enjoy the movies, candy, Cokes, whatever. I ran my clothespin business until I was about nine years old. I had a helper some of the time — a likeable little kid named Eddie Stravitz who lived in the apartment building next door. He was five years younger than I was, only about five years old when he started helping me. We had a lot of fun together while we took care of business (think Little Rascals). I was very happy to run into Eddie many years later, and our friendship was instantly rekindled (which I'll talk about later). One day, I asked the neighborhood grocer if I could deliver groceries for him and, despite the fact that I worked on tips only, I made pretty good tip money. When the launderette opened in 1948, I asked the owners of both the grocery and the launderette if I could split my time between them to deliver for both. They agreed, and I was able to double my pay. I guess I always had a desire for more — to make my way in the world on my own terms.

I only wish that I had the same level of dedication and sense in my schoolwork that I did for making a buck. Back then, I didn't appreciate the importance of education, and I had no concept of what it could do for me. Because of my working-class family background, it wasn't instilled in me at an early age. But I now know how important it is to give kids direction and encourage them to focus on education. I certainly had an intense love of working hard and earning money, even more than I did playing baseball and football with the other kids my age.

That said, I did have my share of fun with the neighborhood kids. One pleasant memory is riding our bikes (mine was borrowed from my older cousin, Myron) almost two miles to watch Jackie Robinson leave his house for Ebbets Field. He was the first African-American baseball player to make it into the major leagues, and we thought he was a God. He was! Jackie didn't have time for us, but we always tried to get him to stop and talk anyway. He'd get into a waiting car and head to the field to play for the Brooklyn Dodgers, a team he dominated from 1947 to 1956, and when Jackie waved at us, we were beyond excited.

Even back then, I'd already started developing "street smarts," or a knack for impressing the right people. At least I thought so. One time, while walking home from playing ball with some friends at the Somers Junior High School schoolyard, we ran into a couple of thugs from "The Paradise Gang." One of its members, a kid named "Nudge" (Irwin was his real name), stopped me and told me that I'd better give him some money or I couldn't pass. When I said "No," Nudge literally nudged me. At which point my friends promptly ran away. Undeterred, I told him "No!" a second time and he proceeded to punch me in the face. I was so outraged, that I instinctively punched him back, and we wound up getting into a full-fledged fight. When the dust settled, I apparently wound up breaking his nose. Oops. His friends took him to Beth-El Hospital and I promptly ran home, where I stayed for the next few days. I'd heard from friends that Nudge wanted to kill me, so I didn't leave my apartment. But when I realized that I couldn't run forever, I finally left the house. Of course, when his friends saw me they commanded me to follow them to their clubroom. So I dutifully went.

When I got there, Nudge was sitting at a card table with a bandage on his nose and two black eyes. He saw me walk in, stood up and immediately began making threats. He then pulled a knife out if his pocket and threw it into the floor right in front of me. I was scared, but I didn't want to let them see me sweat. The truth is that I thought I could beat him again if I had to. Then a strange thing happened: Penny, one of the "leaders" of the gang, interrupted and said, "Hey guys, why don't we all shake hands." And guess what? We did. He also went on to say that he liked my style and by the way, would I like to join the gang? "What???!!!"

Wow, what an honor. At least that's what I thought at the time. Partially because I was happy to be alive. In hindsight, though, how foolish I was to be impressed by these characters. I guess I followed like a sheep, trying to act tough when I needed to. It was probably my survival instinct kicking in, but I knew on some level that my destiny was not to stay in that life for very long. I had dreams and greater visions and hopes, and although I didn't know where to look next, I was excited about where life would lead me. A few of the gang members were smart enough to eventually fight their way out, but most wound up in jail or dead. Being part of the gang didn't really provide any extra benefit to me, except for the fact that I wasn't picked on by the neighborhood guys anymore.

We hung out at Marge's Candy Store or the clubroom, sang, danced, looked for fights, and impressed ourselves by thinking we were part of bigger gang called "Fulton Rockaway." One night, we jumped on the back of fruit trucks to fight a rival gang in another neighborhood (think West Side Story). Fight and hang out, hang out and fight. Sing, dance, fight some more — what a life. Stupid. Looking back, I sometimes wonder if it would have made any difference if my parents had been more educated or if they had demanded that I get an education and become a doctor, lawyer or something, like many of the other Jewish parents in the area.

My parents were such good people, busy trying to make their way and take care of their responsibilities, but if they had pushed me in some direction — any direction — I wonder how/if things might have turned out differently. Maybe I would have been more successful than I am now and moved ahead in life a lot sooner. Or maybe not having the impetus to push myself, perhaps I wouldn't have ever developed the drive and ambition that I did. I'm sure everyone has these thoughts to a certain degree; in any event, they never discouraged me and always made me feel that I could do anything. For that, I'll always be grateful to them for unconditionally loving me and teaching me, by example, to work hard and to always treat people the way I'd like to be treated. Thanks, Mom and Dad, for the many valuable lessons and for teaching me to have no fear and make me feel like I was capable of anything.

> **Mini-Lesson:** *I guess you could say that this is when the start of my real education began. The whole episode taught me that sticking up for oneself (by force if necessary) was a requirement in life, especially in my neck of the woods. Fighting cancer in my world was no different—one must dig deep and begin the fight for and of your life. Not so different than being pushed around by a bunch of local thugs. You have to fight back, and you learn quickly if you truly want to survive. A true entrepreneur can have no fear.*

January 1950 - Brooklyn, New York

As is tradition with many young Jewish boys, I was told that I had to attend Hebrew School for the rest of my life (or at least it felt that way). Classes began at age eight and continued through age thirteen. Instruction was intense, and the goal was to learn my haftorah for my Bar Mitzvah. I faithfully attended class each day after school for two hours, studying with Rabbi Green. He praised my singing voice and encouraged me to consider what my grandfather had planned for my future: to become a cantor, to sing at temple for a living and as my vocation. Obviously, I didn't pursue this for my career, though I have always enjoyed singing very much and still do it at the drop of a hat.

My thirteenth birthday and Bar Mitzvah approached, but unlike some of my peers, my family did not have much money, so a big party at a banquet hall was out of the question. My beloved grandmother suggested we have the ceremony and party right in our apartment. She got my parents excited about hosting the two-day event, as she was a marvelous cook and a gracious hostess. That Saturday after the religious service in temple and through Sunday, my house was filled from early in the morning until late at night with family and friends who came to wish me great success in my life. I remember receiving a fountain pen and the traditional money gifts ranging from $1 to $18 (a Jewish tradition).

My Bar Mitzvah was a wonderful event and a memory I will never forget. We were poor, and everyone knew we were poor. But even though we weren't able to do things that other people were able to do, what a great party my family threw for me that weekend. I felt rich in all the ways that count. When I look back on that memory, there is great joy and satisfaction in being able to say, "Oh my God, look at me now." To this day I am still sometimes in awe of what I am capable of doing. On that day I sang a song to my mom and grandmother — their favorite called, "My Yiddish Mama." Even now, I get teary as I recall the words: "Yiddish mama, I miss you more than ever…now."

A very short time after my low budget but amazing Bar Mitzvah, my beloved grandmother Sara Butler passed away from cancer. I guess she held on, waiting for the special day when she could shine for her grandson; showing our guests how much she loved me, with her outstanding cooking and bright smile. And boy did she. She made all our guests feel welcome, and even though she never even left the kitchen during the whole party, she was smiling and laughing through-out the whole celebration with a gracious warm welcome for everyone. My grandmother was one of the great women in my life who always taught me by example to do for others and to treat people the way you want to be treated. Thanks Bub.

My early years of school didn't inspire me or expose me to any educational role models. Being part of the gang still left time to work at odd jobs. One day when I was fifteen I decided to quit school altogether, but I was informed by a truant officer that it was mandatory that I attend at least some kind of school. I sought out the advice of two people who were close to me — one was Uncle Izzy, who lived around the corner on 96th Street. He worked for the Daily Mirror, a New York newspaper, and set type for a living. He was a good guy. The other was my cousin Hesh Breger, the nicest guy in the world, who worked as a printer for the U.S. Government. I was highly influenced by these two men that I liked and respected. They both advised me to go to the New York School of Printing, a real trade school, and I decided to follow their advice.

So off I went to Manhattan every day by train, getting off at the Empire State Building — 34th Street stop. I learned the word "straphanger". At the trade school, there were a lot of dropouts just like me — tough and stupid. Several months into my time at printing school, five Italian kids from Washington Heights jumped me in the men's room. When I got home and tried to get my pals in the Paradise Gang to go to Washington Heights with me and get even, they weren't in the least bit interested. So I quit the gang and never returned to Printing School.

I enrolled in Continuation School (which at that time was a place to park unruly students — basically one step before jail) on Flatbus Avenue. Of course, this school was also filled with dropouts. There were typing classes and more typing classes, which I basically had no choice but to take (who knew that someone would invent the computer and that it would come in so handy). Also during this time, I worked for A.S. Beck Shoes on Fifth Avenue as a stock boy, while trying to learn how to be a salesman. I was grateful to Allen Schwartz and his father, Mac, for giving me experience working in their Bensonhurst ladies shoe store in Brooklyn for a couple of days, as A.S. Beck hired me right away due to my experience at the Schwartz's store (illustrating that all experience can be good experience, as you never know what will wind up being helpful to you down the road). It was there that I got my first taste of office politics.

When Mr. Kay the boss man was out, the assistant manager Mr. Delmaster took over. Mr. Delmaster was also a taskmaster, who pushed people around without a care. Finally, one day while he was in charge, two of his top salespeople couldn't take it anymore so they up and quit. When Mr. Kay returned, none of the other employees would tell him why his top two salespeople were gone. When he asked me, I may have embellished a bit and told him that Delmaster fired them. Mr. Kay scolded Delmaster, but then the next day when Kay went to lunch, I got canned. So much for my printing, typing and shoe sales careers. But it just goes to show you that although you may have a lot of false starts, don't let them get you down. At that time in my life I didn't really understand the importance of having passion, commitment and discipline for your work — this I learned later. But nonetheless, I was accumulating a ton of life experience that would serve me well in the years to come — in more ways than I could've ever imagined.

> **Mini-Lesson:** *Sometimes it's best to keep your mouth shut — some things are just none of your business.*

January 1953

As a couple of spies named Rosenberg were facing execution for treason and the Korean War was ending, I turned sixteen and was searching for job ideas, a way to make money and to support myself. Through the want ads in the paper, I met Jerry Martin. Although I didn't realize it at the time, becoming an employee of this man gave me many life lessons and taught me much about business, ethics and accountability. His ad stated that he was looking for a young salesman willing to learn a new business and travel. When I met with him, he told me that he saw great potential for me to become a top salesman — but maybe he said that to everyone. I was inspired to believe him.

Even back then I subscribed to the adage, "If you think you can, you can," as well as "If you think you are, you are." Jerry had a business based in Vermont and asked me to work for him there. Without even knowing exactly what I'd be doing, I knew that I wanted to go. New England was far away from Brooklyn, which to me was part of the appeal, but not to my parents. I finally convinced my Mom and Dad that I needed this job and promised that I'd come home often. Reluctantly, they agreed. So I proceeded to quit Continuation School by never showing up again.

So I took my first trip was to Burlington, Vermont, where Jerry taught me how it was to be a "tin man" — selling roofing, siding, storm windows and doors. I was to become the new "door knocker" who had all the answers and knew everything. The truth was, I was as naïve as a babe in the woods — I knew nothing and didn't have a clue as to what was really going on. Jerry said that he had some business cards left over from his previous assistant named Eddie Hart and would I mind using his name, since no one knew me up in Vermont anyway? He assured me that when those cards ran out, I'd get my own. The cards never ran out. I'd soon learn that this was Jerry's style.

I'd go into a neighborhood and knock on doors reciting the canned pitch he taught me. It went something like "…my father, Mr. John Hart, owns an aluminum siding company and he sent me out with Mr. Martin, the regional sales manager so I could learn the business from the ground up." I'd then inform them that I had chosen their home to be used as a model house for a local advertising campaign and if they agreed, they could get their home siding job completed for free, or practically free, as every sale we received from their photograph, would earn them up to $200.

I would offer to make an appointment for that evening for them to meet with Mr. Martin, who would have the ultimate say in whether or not their house would be "chosen" for use in future ads. Now it's not difficult for ten or more houses to be done, we'd say, which would make their job free. In fact, they could even make an additional profit. They'd almost always say yes, and when Mr. Martin showed up he was such a fantastic salesman, that out of every 10 appointments, he'd close around 7. Imagine those statistics…seven out of ten potential customers sold. Wow. That's impressive. For me, the job training was as close as it gets to getting an MBA in the sales world.

In each town, he would first go to the Chief of Police and offer him free siding for his home. He'd say that he was going into business locally and all he wanted in exchange was a good recommendation. He'd give the Chief the best-quality job so when people called, he would tell them, "Jerry Martin is a great guy who does a really good job." The customers bought, and Jerry set up FHA (Federal Housing Authority) loans so he could get paid right away. Everyone was happy. I know I was. I was earning over $200 a week, an absolute fortune at that time — at least for me. When I came home for a visit and told my Dad my weekly earnings, he thought I was robbing banks, since his salary was only about half that amount. Turns out he wasn't that far off.

Life was good. Jerry had an open spot and I convinced my childhood friend, Bob Soll, who had also dropped out of high school to come join me in Vermont. I'll always be thankful for his willingness to leave his dad's lighting and glass factory and join me in the adventures of being a tin man. I was thrilled to have my buddy there with me. We lived in a small but clean local motel, and Jerry gave us the use of his car, though neither of us had a driver's license yet. Fortunately we both knew how to drive and we had a wild time. Jerry trained us to sell siding and taught us tips on life, while we drove around trying to pick up girls in his '53 Cadillac convertible. He told us that the trick was to take the car to a drive-in, order coffee, and when the girls brought the tray, take a sip of coffee and quickly spit it out saying it's wasn't so good that day. We were to then ask for the check, pay the bill, leave a $5 tip and drive away. When we returned the next day, he told us that the girls would all want to go out with us. Guess what? It worked.

Bob and I had a great time in Montpelier, Vermont, and our adventures forever changed my views of business and selling. We didn't get paid often, but we were making more than we ever had, so we felt rich. One day we were driving around town and we saw the installation men at one of our houses that Jerry specifically told us had not closed. When we mentioned it to Jerry, he told us that someone else had brought in the sale. But that wasn't true. We caught him in a lie, and unfortunately it was never the same again. He knew we were onto him, and the next time we all went back to Brooklyn, Bob and I quit our tin man jobs. We had just turned seventeen years old.

A few days later, Jerry's wife, Gladys, called and told me to get out of town. Federal agents had just come to their home to take Jerry away and they were coming to get me too. Shocked, I asked her why, and she explained that although Jerry had gotten FHA money, he had not put the necessary quality of siding on any of the houses other than the Chief of Police's. Many people complained, and the law finally caught up with him. I told my Mom the news Gladys had shared, and we were both very scared, but then I had a great idea (or at least I thought so). I decided to join the Army so they wouldn't find me. So I went down to the enlisting offices on Pitkin Avenue in Brooklyn, then raced home to have my reluctant mother sign the enlistment papers, since I was just seventeen. I raced back with the papers and before I had a chance to change my mind, `I boarded the bus to Fort Dix, New Jersey, and committed the next three years of my life to Uncle Sam.

I found out that while I was en route to Fort Dix, Federal Agents did in fact come to my house looking for me. When my mother told them I'd joined the Army they told her that was plenty of punishment for a kid who apparently hadn't known much about the scam Jerry Martin had been running for years. To my mother's relief, the agents were satisfied with what she told them, and they left. There was a newspaper story that came out a few days later on Jerry's scam and subsequent imprisonment. He got twenty years in a state penitentiary, and I heard that he ultimately died in prison. Life is full of narrow escapes and I was very lucky that this was one of mine. Jerry wasn't so lucky, but I guess he had it coming. I had a lot of time to think on that bus ride. Although I'll always look back fondly on my 'tin man' days, when I got a chance to get out of Brooklyn, earn some money and get a taste of what it feels like to close a deal (which became addictive), an important lesson was not lost on me: there are no shortcuts and there is no easy way to the top.

■ Life Lesson 2: There Are No Shortcuts.

Although I always had a strong work ethic and an entrepreneurial streak that was clearly evident even at 6 years old (when I started my clothespin business), it did take me some time to fully understand that it takes hard work and perseverance to achieve, and most importantly, SUSTAIN long-term gains.

Sure, I was tempted to take shortcuts — hanging out at Marge's Candy store and getting into trouble with the local bullies seemed a heck of a lot easier than going to school or struggling at various jobs. But you know what? The type of "success" gained from the quick-fix approach usually doesn't last. If you can't back up your big talk with action and deliver the goods, eventually you will get found out and it will all come crashing down around you. There is no substitute for good, old-fashioned, hard work. Just ask "Jerry the Tin Man."

CHAPTER THREE
Beyond Brooklyn

LIFE LESSON #3...

*TO BE ENTHUSIASTIC, YOU GOTTA
ACT ENTHUSIASTIC*

---

*"The only limit to our realization of tomorrow
will be our doubts of today."*
- Franklin Delano Roosevelt

1953 - Fort Dix, New Jersey

A new world opened for me in the Army. When they asked me which area I was interested in, for some reason I told them I that I wanted to be an M.P. — a member of the Military Police. I knew those guys got respect, and carried a big stick. I guess that appealed to me. I was told that I would have to travel to Augusta, Georgia to receive training, and I happily agreed. My trip to Georgia was an experience of a lifetime. It was January, and I considered it my birthday present. But my very first airplane ride ever was in a tiny twelve- passenger plane flying from New Jersey to Georgia through horrible weather the entire flight. I wound up getting my birthday present in the form of those little sickness bags provided. I arrived in Fort Gordon, Georgia for training and got my first exposure to the South. The Georgia folk were very hospitable.

I saw myself becoming a police officer, and I knew I could handle the training and do well. But in addition to going through tough physical and mental training, I also had to go through a series of "life tests" as well. They cut off all my hair, put me in a room with forty-eight men, gave me a uniform, a blanket and a bunk. The problem was that I was still a tough Brooklyn punk — a wise guy who thought I could beat it all. Boy, did the Army teach me a few things. Every time I mouthed off to a Sergeant (or anyone for that matter), they found another grease pit for me to dig or a latrine to clean with MY toothbrush. Let's just say I wound up spending a LOT of money on new toothbrushes.

One night in the barracks I was awoken by the sound of something (or someone) falling into my bunk. It seemed a 6'3" fellow serviceman from Alabama named Johnson for some reason (maybe it had something to do with my smart mouth) decided that I shouldn't live anymore. He took a fold-up shovel (known as an entrenching tool) and promptly tried to take my head off. Fortunately, three things were in my favor: 1-Johnson was stupid, 2- I was on the bottom bunk, so he couldn't swing the shovel properly, and 3-Bernard Dugat, better known as Tex, was awake and witnessed what was basically an attempted murder, and knocked Johnson off his feet and into my bed. I quickly jumped out of my bunk, and with that, it seemed like everyone in the barracks woke up, the lights flew on and the mass fighting began.

Turned out that my skirmishes on the streets of Brooklyn streets actually paid off. That with the combat and military police training I'd gotten so far, made me pretty good at defending myself. Private Johnson landed in the hospital for two weeks, and I realized the value and need for friendship and how the buddy system worked. Tex and I became fast friends. I felt lucky. He was a true Texan, a real character who was a rodeo rider and an oil field worker. Tex loved to play guitar and sang country music. I also developed a relationship with Sergeant Williams, a masterful hand-to-hand combat instructor. Sergeant Williams introduced me to Aikido and Tai Chi. Slowly but surely, my world started to expand and my view of life began to extend beyond the streets of Brooklyn. I had to learn fast and adapt quickly, but once I got a taste, I jumped in and didn't look back.

> **Mini-Lesson:** *It pays to make friends so that you have someone to watch your back and "care enough." It has always worked for me.*

After training, I was sent overseas to Germany as an official member of the Military Police. Becoming an MP was the first real goal that I set my sights on and achieved (despite a few bumps along the way), and it was a major milestone for me. It gave me the confidence to go even further. I wanted to make something more of myself. I had drive and ambition. I wanted to keep growing and learning and getting better. I didn't want to be a private the rest of my life. But I found out that I couldn't grow in rank as quickly as I wanted. I apparently would need to be in the service of the Military Police for at least 4 years to even be considered for a NCO (non-commissioned officer) rank. That was way too long for me.

Although I was frustrated, I did some investigating and found out that I could move up faster by moving to a different unit. So what did I do? I decided to try out for the band, of course. That's right, all thanks to my Aunt Syd. You see she and her husband, Calichio Caccioppo (Uncle Charlie), owned a music school, and were also very talented musicians themselves. They basically made it mandatory for all of the kids in the family to play an instrument. That's how I picked up the clarinet, and I'll always be grateful for their musical influence. At thirteen, I even played with an orchestra at the Brooklyn Academy of Music. Wow, a regular Benny Goodman!

Although I wasn't a very talented musician, I played loud and showed great enthusiasm. It now came in handy. I was accepted into the 364th Military Band and was happily transferred, along with my buddy and fellow clarinet player, Tex. We spent the balance of our European military time (almost two years) in Germany traveling with the band, playing marching songs, polkas and "oom-pah-pah" music all over the country as official military guests. I eventually became one of the band leaders. We often travelled on TDY (temporary duty assignment), and I was able to visit Denmark, Italy, and England, both with and without the band.

All in all, Europe was a fun, rewarding, educational time of my life that I'll always remember with smiles. Upon returning to the United States, I still had the better part of a year to serve in the Army. I was next sent to Colorado Springs, Colorado, and, since there wasn't exactly an opening for a Sergeant Band Director there, I was asked to work in the hospital at Fort Carson. I told them it was questionable as to whether I'd be able to handle the job. After being sent to medical and surgical technician training school, where I asked to leave the room a lot to throw up, I miraculously got my diploma and was put on the night shift at the hospital. I learned quickly how to give pills and shots really well. The queasiness factor decreased, and I managed to get six hours of sleep each morning after my shift.

I also finally got a car of my own — a 1941 Nash with a running board. It never needed much gas, but I had to stop every twenty miles to put in oil, always keeping a case in the trunk for emergencies. When I shut the car off, the oil cap would hit the hood and raise it, and smoke would come out of the engine. I learned not to park too close to where I was headed, slightly embarrassed of my car. I got a job off base in a men's clothing store working around thirty hours a week. I had taken and passed the GED (High School Equivalent) test while I was stationed in Europe, so I was able to take classes in English and Psychology at Colorado University extension school for six months. At long last, I finally understood the meaning and importance of pursuing an education.

One night I went to the NCO club to meet some buddies of mine for dinner and drinks. An emergency prevented them from showing up, however, I decided to stay after I spied this beautiful girl sitting two tables away with 3 guys and 4 other gals. I asked her to dance and she agreed. While we were dancing, I knew that something rocked me about this shy, innocent girl. Her name was Fritzie Mogford. She was from Texas and currently living in Colorado Springs while studying to be an X-ray Technician. I'd never heard of a name like hers before, and she explained that she was the fourth daughter, and her dad's name was Fritz, so it was just her luck to be called Fritzie. I knew she was going to be mine, so I asked her that night to marry me. She told me I was crazy, and I agreed. We dated from that moment on from April to July, dancing almost every date except for movie night.

> **Mini-Lesson:** *Allow yourself to get carried away. Don't let being shy stop you from opening the door to life. Life is good, but you have to walk through that door to go out and get it. Not fully expressing your feelings is akin to winking at a girl in the dark — why bother?*

We were great together, and she agreed to visit New York with me at the end of June for the wedding of a childhood friend, Judy Aronoff, who has always been like a sister to me. Fritzie and I arrived in New York, and I believe she was in a state of shock the entire time. I think it started with my mom's first words to her at Idlewild Airport: "Welcome to New York. See, we don't have horns." The wedding was at the Belle Harbor Jewish Center on Long Island — a black-tie affair with an entirely Jewish guest list. It was certainly a new experience for Fritzie, a farm girl from Texas who had never been to a fancy event like that before, where everyone was dressed to the nines. I was in uniform, and Fritzie was wearing a simple dress. We both felt out of place so we left early and I took her to my home away from home in Brooklyn — Nathan's in Coney Island. The hot dogs and rides were all great fun, but I guess for someone who had never seen New York before, Fritzie was so overwhelmed by the day's events that you'd think I had taken her to outer space.

One week after arriving in New York, Fritzie and I decided to get married. After four rabbis refused, we finally found one in Roslyn, Long Island, who would help us. Fortunately the Rabbi was in the military as a chaplain. He explained that the other orthodox and reformed Rabbis refused to marry us because they didn't want mixed marriages in the Jewish faith and they figured we would just go away and change our minds. But one thing that we did know was that we had a desire and a need to be in each other's lives and nobody was going to change that. I bought a ring for Fritzie, and though it wasn't much, it wasn't a cigar wrapper either. I didn't fully realize it then, but I surely do now: Fritzie Mogford Levine was the best thing that ever happened to me.

I think our families were in shock. Actually I hadn't even met her family yet. Fritzie and I exchanged wedding vows on Independence Day, the Fourth of July in 1957, just 4 months after we met at the NCO club. I was grateful to have Bob Soll and his new wife, as well as my Pop there with us. It was not like any wedding we had ever been to then or since. My Dad took the whole family (all seven of us) to dinner at a restaurant on Eastern Parkway in Brooklyn to celebrate. Talk about a small wedding. But that was okay with us. We were happy and in love.

However, there was someone who wasn't exactly happy for us. The lucky man from Kiev, Shia Gershonowitz — my grandfather, Sam Levine — who was by now a rabbi. When I married Fritzie, the daughter of a

Mormon mother and a Baptist father, he was very unhappy, to say the least. He felt that I was betraying our faith and breaking an important tradition. He let me know how he felt about my mixed marriage by simply never speaking to me — ever again. He even sat *shiva* for me, the Jewish tradition of mourning a loved one's passing. That's when I really knew that I was dead to him. It was a very sad experience for Fritzie and I, but nothing could be done about it. We chose to have a life together, and that was that.

> **Mini-Lesson:** *Life is about choices. They are not always easy and people you love and care about may not agree with them, but that goes with the territory. I certainly never regretted my choice to marry Fritzie, but I believe that I would've always regretted caving into my grandfather's wishes to NOT marry her.*

I took Fritzie on a honeymoon we would never forget. I had gotten rid of the old Nash in Colorado, along with all of its oil and hood problems. As soon as I got to New York, I bought a used car. I was thrilled that the dealer gave me such a good price, and figured it was because I was in the Army and about to get married. I made reservations at the Fallsview Hotel in the Catskills, and after our small family dinner, we drove through Manhattan onto the West Side Highway toward the George Washington Bridge, planning to make it up there before evening.

Well, we never made it. That great buy of a car broke down at 96th Street on the West Side Highway. We called a tow truck that took the car to a garage and dropped us off at a nearby hotel on 45th Street called The Paramount. The hotel room had a saggy mattress and was just little bit larger than a closet. There was no air conditioning either. We wound up spending the week trying to get our money back from the Fallsview Hotel as well as the car dealer. We lost one and won one, but we survived — we were in love. My new bride and I hung out in New York City, went to a lot of movies, a Broadway show, and ate from a lot of food vendors. Even though it wasn't exactly what we had planned, we saw lots of "fireworks," and thoroughly enjoyed being newlyweds and beginning our new life together.

The following week, I was due back in Colorado to report for duty. Fritzie stayed with my Mom and Dad since I had four months left in the service and she had a job opportunity in Brooklyn. We figured that it would only be for a short time, and it would all be for the best. Boy were we wrong. So Fritzie worked as an X-ray technician at Beth-El Hospital while I went back to Fort Carson, Colorado. While there, I took a long weekend to Texas to finally meet Fritzie's family. The hospitality and warmth was great — Fritzie's family was full of great people of simple means. My father-in-law Fritz let me know immediately that he had someone for me to meet, a potato farmer, "who was also a Jew." He introduced me as his new son-in-law, "Lee-Vine." We had a good laugh, his friend was a good guy, and my father-in-law called me "Lee-Vine" for the rest of his life.

But I missed my wife. During this time Fritzie also discovered that she was pregnant. Although we were thrilled, time went by even more slowly in the Army, and the frustration of not seeing my wife was increasing. I found myself often getting into trouble and losing stripes for speaking out of turn. In the military that is not tolerated. It was tough being so far away from her, even though we called each other almost every night from Colorado to Brooklyn (that is, until the phone bill arrived, and it was out of this world). So we began writing letters. I realize now that newlyweds should not be apart and Fritzie probably should have joined me in Colorado instead of enduring the culture shock of living with my parents in Brooklyn.

In the meantime, due to my repeated run-ins with the military authority, I was moved from hospital duty and put on ping-pong duty at the Recreation Center. It was a tough job: waking at 7 a.m., opening the room, keeping an eye on the Coke machine and the ping-pong table until 4 p.m. Whether I liked it or not, I became a pretty good ping pong player (I still am to this day and have had a ping pong table in the house for the last 35 years). This plum assignment gave me more time to work downtown at Pop's clothing store, but more importantly, it allowed me the chance to give some serious thought to my future, especially now that I would have a family to support, and I knew that I couldn't make a living playing ping pong.

My four months were finally up and the Army tried to convince me to re-enlist. Not a chance. I took my Honorable Discharge, boarded a train with everything I owned in two duffel bags and headed back to Brooklyn. I felt like the luckiest guy in the world. The train stopped in Chicago, and I was told that there would be a 24-hour delay to New York. This was unacceptable to me — my wife and family were waiting, and my patience was gone. I left my bags on the train and took a bus to the airport, boarded a plane and flew into the waiting arms of my wife and parents. With no more Uncle Sam to feed and clothe and house me, not to mention the $400 combined Army and income from Pop's store, it was time to get serious about finding work.

A couple of days after returning to New York, I went to Penn Station to retrieve my duffel bags and was questioned by the police as to why I switched my train ticket in Chicago to a plane ticket. I explained that I couldn't wait to get home and asked why they cared. I had not seen the newspaper, so I wasn't aware that the train I was to be on had derailed, killing one person and injuring many others. I realized that I really was one lucky son-of-a-gun. God was certainly watching over me that day; and he has been every day of my life since.

Life Lesson 3: To Be Enthusiastic, You Gotta Act Enthusiastic.

I have always maintained that more than half the battle in life is having a positive attitude. No, I wasn't the best clarinet player in the world (or even in Brooklyn for that matter), but I played loud and proud and enjoyed myself. That got me into the Army band and enabled me to advance rank faster than I would have otherwise. I wanted to move forward and I wasn't going to let anyone or anything slow me down. There was a wall, and I was determined to find a way around it, over it, under it, or through it.

This is very different from looking for a shortcut. I didn't want to avoid hard work, but I did want to focus on ways that I could see some concrete progress. Setting a small or medium-sized goal and achieving it gave me the confidence to aim even higher next time. Then there's the way I met and married my wife. I knew she was the best thing that ever happened to me and she felt it too, but I was able to win her over with my enthusiasm. She was able to trust her feelings all the more because of how convinced I was. During my trip home to New York, my enthusiasm literally couldn't be contained. I needed to get there faster. Changing my travel plans to accommodate my impatience, not only saved my life, but taught me a valuable lesson: The only path you should follow is your own.

CHAPTER FOUR
Hairstylist To The Stars

LIFE LESSON #4...

IF YOU DO NOTHING, YOU GET NOTHING

"How far that little candle throws his beam, so shines a
good deed in a weary world."
— William Shakespeare

---

*A*fter a few weeks back in New York trying to figure out what to do next and how to support my growing family, I was excited to tell Fritzie that I wanted to be a hairstylist. That's right. She was surprised (to say the least), but when I explained to her my rationale, she agreed and fully supported my idea. I chose the profession for a couple of reasons. First of all there were only 6 months of school required, and with the baby on the way in about 4 months, that seemed doable. But even more importantly, when I was young, my Aunt Syd and Uncle Charlie would let me sleep over their house on occasional weekends. They'd take me to Sunday luncheons at the Caccioppo house.

Uncle Charlie's four brothers were always there, and they always loved to brag to each other. The most boastful brother was Casper who called himself the "The Best Hairstylist in the World." Maybe he was, maybe he wasn't. All I knew was that he lived in a big, beautiful house in Brooklyn, drove a new Cadillac and dressed like he just stepped out of Bergdorf Goodman's. Casper the friendly hairstylist always had money in his pocket for everything. Is there anything else in life, I thought? He had it all. As a kid, I was impressed and I never forgot. At my wonderful adopted Italian family's house, I'd sit on Nana Caccioppo's lap and she would fondly call me her "ruffiano" (ruffian). I have lots of wonderful memories there.

Mini-Lesson: *It's always about family.*

I also recalled that when I graduated from the 6th grade a classmate's father, Mr. Murray, wrote in my yearbook: "Be Independent!" He had been my mom's hairstylist when I was young. He was a very good man with a tremendous generosity of spirit, who was always doing good deeds. Mr. Murray impressed me, and his words echoed in my brain all my life. So, I was off to be a hairstylist. My father thought I was turning into a "fag," which was the way of thinking back then, but nothing was further from the truth (not that there's anything wrong with that). I just wanted to make a lot of money, drive a nice car, have a great house filled with beautiful things, live great and be popular. Doesn't everybody?

Mini-Lesson: *Believe in who you want to be.*

So I began my training at the Wilfred Academy Beauty School in New York City on Broadway and 51st Street right next door to Lindy's Restaurant. I was pleased when the owner told me that tuition would be free under the G.I. Bill. Now that the money was covered, I would begin classes in January. Fritzie and I wanted our own apartment so we quickly moved into an apartment in Brooklyn on East 15th Street off Kings Highway in the heart of Flatbush. It was next to the train station and we had to bang on the pipes for heat. We were always freezing and had to dress for bed in turtlenecks, socks, sweatpants and lots of blankets. But we were happy.

I needed money for rent and food so I took a job during the day with Fuller Brush in door-to-door sales. I sold a lot of toothbrushes in my territory of the Bensonhurst section of Brooklyn. I remember so well that whenever it got slow and sales weren't good, I could go to Perry Como's mother. She lived in the area, and I could always count on her to buy something from me. Thank you, marvelous Mrs. Como, wherever you are. What a talent your son brought to the world. That job wasn't really enough to live on, so I took a job in Abrams Carriage and Children's Furniture Store to supplement my income. I worked Fuller Brush from Monday to Friday, Wilfred Academy on Tuesday, Thursday, and Friday nights and at the furniture store on weekends. One main reason I took the job at the furniture store was so I could buy my new baby things at a discount and get paid by the hour.

On March 17, 1958, St. Patrick's Day, our first son was born. Some of my friends asked why we didn't name him Patrick, and I said that he'd have a helluva time explaining away the name Patrick Levine — it just didn't work. We named him after my grandmother, Sara, and called him Steven

Lee (Jewish tradition is that you use the first letter of the deceased whom you wish to honor). Fritzie wanted Lee as the middle name because that's how she first knew me. My Army buddies had shortened my last name of Levine to 'Lee,' and of course, I'm still called "Uncle Lee" by all of Fritzie's family. The luck of the Irish arrived that day with Steve.

Anyway, with a child, the choice was pretty clear that I'd have to go to school for eighteen months at night - or I could switch over to days, get a night job and move back in with my parents. They wanted us with them so badly, and I think we made the right decision when we moved back to their apartment on Rockaway Parkway. It worked out great for a while. They were so happy watching Steve grow and babysitting while I took in hairstyling customers in our bedroom. I cut hair, colored and shampooed in local shops on the weekend while finishing school.

During my time at Wilfred Academy, I liked to eat and study at Taffernetti's Restaurant on Broadway. One day, I walked in, wearing my white smock, carrying some books, and I headed toward an empty table. As I walked by a table of five guys, one wise guy said, "Look at the fag hairstylist!" They all chimed in, laughing, and one of them knocked my books to the floor. I asked him to pick them up, and he laughed some more and pushed me. As he pushed, I pulled. I had a twenty second fight with five guys. I think I got the better of them, because they were seated and I was standing. I picked up my books and left the restaurant, never to return. When I shared the story with my school friend Sal, he told me he had seen it in the newspaper. Apparently, a columnist had gotten wind of it and wrote it up, with the headline: "Don't Mess with Your Hairstylist." For a few years I carried that article around with me as a badge of honor.

> **Mini-Lesson: *Don't mess with your hairstylist.***

Every year, each graduating class has a contest for the best stylist. Cocky as I was, I told everyone before we graduated from Wilfred not to bother to enter the contest for graduates because I was going to win. Fritzie was my model, and I guess all the practice I got doing my family's hair while

I went to school paid off. I did indeed win, and received a medal, plus a six week apprenticeship at John Fonda's salon. He was the man who really taught me the art of cutting hair. In the 1950s he was one of the premiere names in the world of hairstyling. Leon Amendola, Charles of the Ritz, Robert Fiance, and John Fonda were all known as the best of the best — the Vidal Sassons of their time, if you will.

I quickly took to my craft and started to work in Brooklyn, making $60 to $70 per week plus tips, while getting exposure to people in all walks of life. I'd never realized how much a part of everyday life a hairstylist plays. The relationships formed, the bonds made, the camaraderie with clients — it was all addictive to me. The passion to get better and better at a skill really got into my blood, and I couldn't get enough education. I went to Clairol, L'Oreal, and Rayette schools at night for more certifications, learning more about coloring, permanent waves — really mastering the craft. All the while, I learned about relationships like never before. The truth is I was good — never the most highly skilled or talented, but my personality made up for anything that was missing. This is when I truly started asking the question, *"How Can I Help You?"* on a daily basis and to everyone I encountered.

After a while of living back home with my parents, Fritzie announced that now that I had my hairstyling license, it was time for us to go out on our own again and I agreed. But where to? We decided we wanted to move to Florida. Fritzie had a wealthy aunt named Marie in Miami Shores who we thought we could stay with while we got situated. Turns out she wasn't really interested in having us stay for more than a few days. As I look back, it was probably the saddest day for my parents. We lived with them for almost a year, and now we were going to take their 8 month old baby grandson to Florida. But I have to give them credit, they didn't try to stop us. They let us forge our own path.

We rented a U-Haul, hooked it up to my 1953 red and white four door Plymouth and headed south. I had no job and little money but we did have a dream to win big. We soon found an apartment on S.W. 11th Street in Miami, a one bedroom downstairs unit for $85 a month. Now

I needed to find a job. I never did check into the whole state license thing, and quickly discovered that my New York license was no good in Florida. I would have to take the Florida test to be qualified to work down there. But with a wife and newborn I needed to make money while I waited for my scheduled licensing exam, so I took a job selling shoes for Butler Shoes in Miami. The pay was equivalent to what one received on unemployment, but I'd never collected it before and would not allow myself to now.

It felt like a long wait, but finally, after a few months, I got called to take the Florida Cosmetology Exam. Once again, I brought Fritzie as my model. I didn't know you had to bring two models as part of Florida's requirement of both a manicure and pedicure exam with a different model. I did fine on head and hair exams, both practical and written. When it came to manicure and pedicure, because I didn't bring an additional model, they supplied me with one. She was a 4'8" tall 300-pound black woman with the sweetest face. I watched the girl next to me and tried to follow her example. But when it came time for the pedicure and I took off the lady's shoes, I nearly passed out due to the smell. She hadn't washed her feet in what seemed like years or just had a severe foot odor problem, and I mean severe.

I had to sit on a small bench at her feet and hold my breath as I worked. I exhaled as I went to get a foot bowl as the girl beside me had done. I told her how awful the smell was, and she confirmed that she smelled it six feet away and suggested some 30 or 40 volume peroxide that is used for bleaching hair. I poured it into the foot bath water, but I think I poured too much as her skin started to bleach up. It was very good that she was so large so she couldn't see just how white her feet suddenly got. The instructor gave me a look and a smile, and I knew I passed the test, probably on ingenuity alone. Thank you, fellow student, for the peroxide tip. Sorry about your white feet, nice customer lady. I hope it wasn't permanent.

After passing the test, I quickly got a job at a brand new salon in Coral Gables, but I soon realized that the owner and investor knew nothing about the business , so I didn't see myself staying there long term. One day I took Fritzie and baby Steve for a ride to Miami Beach. I was a man with a plan. I remember it was raining very hard that day when we drove to the famous Fontainebleau Hotel in Miami Beach. I asked Fritzie to wait across the street in the car with Steve while I visited the hotel's hair salon. I parked the car next to the boat dock by the water so they would have something pleasant to look at while they waited.

I walked through the door of the busy salon and met the man who was going to change my life — and my name, forever. I said to that man standing at the front desk, "Hi, my name is Marvin Levine, and I'm a protégé of John Fonda. I'd really like to work here." Buddy Maurice, the salon's owner and manager asked if I had a Florida license, and I happily told him I did. He then said that the next lady who walked through the door for a comb-out was mine. That's the way he tried out stylists. While I waited, I looked around and couldn't believe how busy it was. It seemed like New Year's Eve in there, even though it was an ordinary Wednesday at 4 o'clock in the afternoon. I remember thinking, "This is the place for me — right in the middle of the action."

Buddy seemed an unlikely owner of a Beauty Salon: short, plump and disheveled, with wild hair, big lips and an even bigger cigar-chomping mouth that constantly hollered orders like a drill sergeant, but all of the ladies loved him. I waited up front with the 3 receptionists until finally the moment arrived — a woman who wanted a comb-out walked in. "Hey you, come here," Buddy yelled to me. I walked to an empty chair in between two highly skilled hairstylists — Gary from Philadelphia who dressed like he was going to a Broadway show, and Allyn from New York City, who apparently did the hair of the entire cast of Guys and Dolls.

I stood there looking incredulously at my new customer, who seemed to be the spitting image of Harpo Marx. I asked if I could give her a wash and set, but she told me she only had time for a comb-out. I explained that her hair was very curly and it was raining and humid outside, but she was adamant that she only wanted a comb-out. I couldn't believe that she was asking me to do this for my try-out. I didn't think it would turn out well, but I really, really wanted the job, so I rolled up my sleeves, went to work and did my best. I pulled, stretched, teased, sprayed and prayed.

Twenty minutes later, the sweat was pouring out of me when I finally finished. The woman looked in the mirror and exclaimed, "It looks great!" I stood there in shock because I actually thought she now looked even more like Harpo than when she walked in. The only thing missing was his horn to squeeze. But she was delighted, and I was surprised, but thrilled. It just goes to show you that even if something seems absolutely impossible, if you give it your all, and really try to please (help) someone, you can succeed.

Harpo, I mean my customer, told Buddy Maurice that I was the best, and she wanted me to do her hair every day. Wow! Buddy took me aside and we spoke for a few minutes. He told me that I did a really good job because the customer was very happy, and that he wanted to hire me. Then he asked, "What's your name again?" I told him I was Marvin Levine. He said, "Okay, you'll be Marvin #4" (since he had three Marvins working there already). I thanked him but said that I didn't want to begin my career as Marvin #4. Buddy asked, "Well, what's your middle name?" When I told him it was Walter, he announced, "I dub you M. Walter" and it's stuck ever since.

> **Mini-Lesson:** *Open to change, an optimist sees every situation as an opportunity.*

He told me to show up the next day at 8:30 a.m. I thanked him and left, but I couldn't contain myself. I ran all the way to the car screaming "Yes! Yes! Yes!" and Fritzie and I hugged each other and laughed with joy. I shared the moment with my wife and baby son by celebrating at the A&W Root Beer Stand with hot dogs and, of course, root beer. When we got home, I called the other salon and told them I was leaving their employ effective immediately, as there were no appointments on the books for me yet, and I'd found a more suitable job for myself at the Fontainebleau Hotel.

I started at the salon the next morning and I was extremely busy from the start making many new friends in my new "working family." In the midst of the hustle and bustle, I enjoyed watching the other sixteen stylists work, as it helped give me ideas on how to get better. I truly loved my work and was becoming a pretty good stylist. I got more and more referrals, and it seemed like every day was a holiday. People were in great moods probably because most of the clientele was on vacation, and I quickly began to settle into my new world. Things were good. I was making $300 to $400 a week and we were finally able to buy furniture for the first time.

This was the first time I was exposed to a "moneyed society" and it was quite an adjustment for me. I was a bit intimidated but I met some wonderful women in the salon, both employees and customers, who tried to help me "open my eyes." They told me not be so naïve. "Don't believe everything you hear from customers and believe only half of what you hear from the other stylists," they told me. I took their advice to heart. One day a very sweet, but plain-looking 60-year old woman sat down in my chair. She told me she was originally from Illinois and was now living in California and in Miami with her boyfriend, Jimmy Durante. I said, "Yeah, right." She promised it was the truth, that Jimmy really was her boyfriend. Keeping in mind what I had been told, I didn't believe her, and I continued to work on her hair for an hour. As I was combing her out, I heard a gravelly, distinctive and familiar voice say, "Has anybody seen my girl?" I turned around, and you guessed it: Jimmy Durante — live and in the flesh. I was so delighted and excited. He looked just like he did on television. I asked for his autograph, and he replied in that voice like no other, "Look, Sonny, my autograph's only good on a check." With that, he took out a check and signed across the entire face of it and handed it to me. As he left, he shook my hand and said, "Thanks for making my girl look so beautiful." He was a great guy.

After that experience, I tried to take the advice of the women who tried to protect me less literally. Instead of being automatically cynical and distrustful, I made the choice to believe unless proven otherwise and although I was sometimes fooled, I found that most people were just wonderful and my opportunities expanded exponentially. I had great times and continued to improve my craft. My reputation grew, and I always asked for referrals from each client I met and formed a relationship with.

Mini-Lesson: *Always ask for referrals — nothing helps to grow your business more than the power of relationships.*

Another thing that helped my success was that I genuinely loved what I was doing. If you really love what you do, it gives you a strong inner desire to be the best. The word for it is passion. One of the greatest things about being a hairstylist is the instant gratification it gives you. A woman can go to the dentist and endure awful pain, or to a doctor for surgery, but have to wait to get well. But give her a great hair style or a terrific perm or color, and watch a happy person walk away from your chair. She's ecstatic and positive and ready to take on the world and any problem the day may bring. The feeling of satisfaction you get from creating that transformation is extremely gratifying. When you are truly focused on the needs of your customer, your success will take care of itself. Invoking the mantra "How Can I Help You?" no matter what your profession will get you there.

One day, two stunning ladies were referred to me, the most beautiful women I had ever seen. They could each have easily won Miss America, and it wasn't hard to for me to make them look great. Actually, they made me look good. They told me they were at the hotel with Frank Sinatra. Due to the good job I did on their hair, Frank came and shook my hand and offered me tickets to that night's World Premiere of his latest movie, "Can Can" on 42nd Avenue in Miami Beach. I said, "Are you kidding me? Yes!" The lovely ladies returned with four tickets. I called Fritzie and invited another couple that drove her to the movie theater, while I arranged to meet them all there.

I remember standing outside the theater as everyone was mingling, and at one point I wound up standing next to Frank Sinatra and the two women. Frank turned to me and said, "Thanks kid. You did good." Frank

Sinatra was actually talking to me. Wow! It was our first experience attending a World Premiere movie event, and it turned out to be a wonderful night. The film was good but even better was the fact that we had seats two rows behind Frank. It was quite a feeling. Actually, I don't recall much of the movie, but I do remember the back of Frank Sinatra's head and those of the two ladies whose hair I had done earlier that day.

> **Mini-Lesson:** *You never know what is going to change your life — even for just one day. Always being the best you can be with passion keeps you prepared for those moments whenever they come along.*

After a few months, I met and did the hair of other stars including Phyllis McGuire of the McGuire Sisters, and May Britt who was married to Sammy Davis Jr. at the time. While I was doing May's hair in their hotel suite I told Sammy, who was there with his wife, that when I was younger I went to Ben Masik's Town & Country in Brooklyn to see the Will Mastin Trio (the group he had with his uncle and father). He loved hearing that and we got along great. So much so that he let me sing with him as he was warming up — fun! I also got to "do" the fabulous and funny Lucille Ball. Now that was an experience. Lucy appeared in my chair, put her feet up and said, "Do me." We had a great time, and laughed throughout the whole appointment. I loved Lucy. Her daughter, Luci Arnaz, is now a fellow Westport, Connecticut resident and does wonderful work with charities in the community, continuing her mom's legacy of kindness.

Not all of my encounters with celebrities went as well. One day a lady sat down in my chair and said she was Roberta Peters, an opera singer. My Miami neighbors, Len and Renee were opera fans and had taught me a bit about the art form. Perhaps being a bit full of myself at this point, I tried to impress her. Boy was that a mistake. I showed my ignorance by saying impulsively, "Oh, I have some of your records at home." She replied with a great big smile, "Oh really. Which ones?" I blurted out, "Uh, La Boheme." She frowned and said, "I never made La Boheme." Instead of shutting up, I put another foot in my mouth and said, "Oh, right. It's Madame Butterfly that I have of your albums." What a schmuck! With that, she got up from my chair and asked the receptionist for a different hairstylist. A lesson learned. It wasn't Roberta Peters whose records I had — it was Renata Tebaldi. Ooops. Twenty years later, Roberta Peters became a client of mine of my alarm company. This time I knew enough to keep my mouth shut and be grateful for her business.

A lot of what I got to experience was due to just plain old timing. For example, I parked my car each day at the hotel, as they gave me a special employee rate. One day, Harry Belafonte was coming out of the hotel at the same time my car was delivered. The doorman asked if I wouldn't mind dropping him off at the Eden Rock Hotel next door to the Fontainebleau as two dozen fans were surrounding him and he needed to get away. I asked what he was doing at the hotel, and he said that he'd stopped over to thank Sammy Davis Jr. for doing his show at the Eden Rock. Harry had gotten sick and they couldn't cancel his show in time, so Sammy filled in. It was a two-minute drive that I'll never forget. Life is about timing. What a warm and kind man he was.

I also met a wonderful array of clients who invited Fritzie and I to shows and dinners at the hotel, ladies who sent my wife gifts of things their husbands manufactured like bathing suits, dresses, toys, etc. It was truly an honor to work there and create the relationships I did. I also met the owner of the Fontainebleau , Mr. Ben Novak — quite a character and a great man. He couldn't hear very well and wore a hearing aid — at the time it was the kind you keep in your pocket with a wire to the ear. I watched him reach into his pocket and turn the sound off while certain people were talking to him, usually when they were asking a favor of him. It was so easy to detect and hilarious to watch. He would pretend to listen and then reply, "Let me think it over. I'll get back to you." His family was in the hotel business in the Catskill Mountains in upstate New York, 90 miles from New York City in an area known as the "Borscht Belt." The area was filled with hotels that catered to upper middle class and wealthy Jewish families who liked to escape from the heat of the city for the summer. Each hotel offered food and entertainment of all kinds included in the price of the room.

Mr. Novak's family owned the Laurels Hotel and Country Club on Sacket Lake. It was run by his sister Miriam Spears and sister-in-law Gladys Novak who both became clients of mine in 1959. Like many of my other clients, they were demanding, but I found them easy enough work with, as I loved what I did. They liked me and made me a business proposition I found hard to refuse. If they cleared it with Buddy Maurice would I leave the salon for the summer, to own and run the beauty salon in the Laurels Hotel in the Catskills? My entrepreneurial spirit was waiting for that moment. I didn't even have to think. I instantly said, "Yes! Yes! Yes!" I felt so excited and fortunate.

> **Mini-Lesson:** *People do business with people they like. What's your style?*

I asked Fritzie that evening how she felt about going back to New York for the summer, and she said yes, but only if we could afford it and maintain our independence. I agreed and when I approached Buddy Maurice with the idea, he said "Go for it." He liked me, but he also liked the fact that I said I would return in October. It worked for both of us, since the summer was the slow season down in Miami. I guess I was lucky to be in the right place at the right time with the right goods. The rest of the season brought great joy, and we truly loved living in the Miami area. Fritzie, Steve and I would drive around on Sundays and look at the beautiful homes in Coral Gables, Miami Beach and the islands attached. Fritzie and I agreed that we would live in a home like one of these one day, knowing it would take much effort and hard work to get there. I began to really learn that if you do nothing, you get nothing. Don't forget to dream. It's worth it.

Life Lesson #4 - If You Do Nothing, You Get Nothing:

Whether it was jumping into the hairstyling business, moving my wife and baby to Florida without a job or place to live, randomly walking into the biggest hotel salon in the area for a tryout or changing my name for a job without blinking an eye, you certainly can't say that I didn't try. I was opening my own doors, and the more I tried, the more I learned, all the while adjusting my approach with the incremental information that I was exposed to along the way. Of course, some of my attempts worked out better than others, but that's not the point. The point is that if you stand still and don't even try because you are afraid of making the wrong decision, one thing is for sure — you won't get anywhere.

So take some chances and have enough faith in yourself to realize that even if you make a few wrong turns along the way, eventually you'll figure it out and arrive in a better place. Always be the best you can be, whatever the weather, and don't forget to bring your own sunshine. And finally, always remember, there are no guarantees in life except for one: If you do nothing, you get nothing. And if you do something, you get something. Visualize! Inspire! Think success!

CHAPTER FIVE
The Climb

"Attitude determines altitude."
— Unknown

---

*S*pring arrived, and it was like someone pulled the plug — where did all the customers go after April 1st? I figured there must have been a special going on at a neighboring salon because our business dropped off by about 70%. I asked my fellow stylists what was happening and they said, "That's why we're called snow birds; we head back up north until Thanksgiving." I couldn't believe it. Thank God I was following my 10% saving's rule even back then, which was to save 10% of everything I made and not spend it unless it "rained." You never think of saving for a rainy day when the sun is shining and the money just keeps flowing in. But anything can happen (and it usually does).

> **Mini-Lesson:** *The Levine 10% Rule says to put 10% of whatever is in your pocket into a jar, every day. When you have $1000 saved up, invest it. (I always suggest putting it into an SSS bond — sewers, streets and schools. Not only does it help build the infrastructure of the world, but it's a safe bet — these are things the world is always going to need.)*

I had befriended Dominick Marchetta, a fellow stylist who also had new ideas about the salon business. He was a handsome bachelor who had a tendency to goof around. For instance, working in a Speedo with a brush and comb sticking out at his hip. Of course, the women loved him. They thought he was crazy but wonderful (and they were right on both counts). I asked Dominick if he was doing anything for the summer and he said that he had no firm plans. I suggested he come to work with me up in the Catskills. He had four years more experience than I did and I thought I'd need the help. He would only agree to join me if I made him a partner, and I agreed to his terms. We shook hands and we were off.

On May 1st, Fritzie, Steve and I headed north, stopping in Brooklyn where we visited my parents for a few days. My grandfather, "Pop," asked us if we would consider taking a larger bungalow in the Catskills so he could join us for the summer. It would give him a chance to spend some time with his great-grandson Steve, and allow him to get away from my mom (his daughter) who he said was "driving him nuts." We happily agreed. Fritzie and I loved Pop so much and we wanted him to develop a relationship with our baby boy. Not to mention, it also gave us an excuse to get a nicer bungalow. So we proceeded on to Sacket Lake laughing with joy and excitement.

> **Mini-Lesson:** *When you start a journey, you gotta take some risks.*

When we got there we scoped out the hotel and beauty salon. It definitely needed some work. But it was nothing that a little carpentry, a few beauty supplies and new carpeting couldn't fix. But before we started on the renovations, Fritzie and I went looking for a new home. Across the street from the hotel was Sondack's Bungalow Colony, where we cut a deal on a great 3 ½ room bungalow for the Summer. It had one bedroom for Pop and the master bedroom for Fritzie and I plus Steve's crib. There was a nice little kitchen with a small screened porch to have our meals. With some creative bartering — I agreed to do Mrs. Sondack's hair at a reduced price — we got a great rate for the summer. To us it was Heaven in the Catskills.

I left Fritzie, Pop and Steve with a kiss each morning and did my thing at the beauty salon. The setting in the hotel was perfect - I would drive right through the main entrance in my stylish red and white Plymouth, up to the guard at the gate who would wave me through. I'd cruise up to the beautiful hotel lobby entrance, a gorgeous lake was on the right, offering swimming, boating, water skiing, and right at the front was the beauty salon. I was happy to be alive. I ordered new signs, and since D came before W alphabetically, we decided to call it Dominick and M.Walter Hairstylists. And in small letters underneath, was "From the Fontainebleau Hotel, Miami Beach." I guess it worked because from Memorial Day to Labor Day we were so busy that we had to hire two more stylists and three shampoo and manicure girls. Wow. We learned, used and taught the question of *"How Can I Help You?"* and it paid off.

We settled down into our new salon playing Frank Sinatra and Sammy Davis, Jr. music on the stereo all day, singing, swinging and doing hair. It was bliss in the Borscht Belt. In addition to the hotel guests, we developed a large clientele from other bungalow colonies and businesses in the area. That is after we took care of the guard at the gate. He allowed our customers to come in without being hassled — all they had to do was say, "We're going to the Beauty Salon," and they were in.

It was during that time that an English lady with a charming accent came into the salon and we got to talking. She gave me some advice that has stayed with me to this day. After chatting for a short time, she said in the nicest way possible "Your problem is that you don't speak correctly. You sound like you come from the streets of Brooklyn," to which I jauntily replied, "That's because I do." In her proper British elocution, she looked into my eyes and asked me earnestly, "My boy, do you have any idea how to speak properly?" I answered, "Uh, yeah." She shook her head and corrected me. "The correct answer is yes."

Realizing that she had a point, I sheepishly asked her, "So how do I learn to speak proper English like you do?" She proceeded to spend the rest of the afternoon patiently teaching me how to enunciate my words slowly and correctly. I never forgot that tutoring session and I'll always appreciate it. With her help and my continued effort, my thick Brooklyn accent became milder and much less obvious. I finally understood that even if you have great things to say, if you don't come across as credible no one will listen to you.

> **Mini-Lesson:** *Try to learn and grow daily. Give of yourself, show acceptance of everyone you meet and watch the magic happen.*

We met and developed relationships with many of the comedians, singers and entertainers who performed at the hotel. I got to do their hair and see their shows. Sometimes we would even hang out with them before or after their performances. It was an amazing experience. I was having fun, business was great and my family was happy and healthy, and we found out that we were pregnant again. Things were good. I got to meet and do hair for Leslie Uggams, who was a child star of 15 at the time. She was a great kid with a terrific attitude and happily sang along with us to the Sinatra and Sammy Davis, Jr. tunes we played at the shop.

That is until one day in August, when one of the children at the bungalow colony got his toy stuck in a tree. He asked Pop, who was watching the children play, to get up from his chair and get the toy. Pop happily obliged, reaching up to pull the toy out of the tree. All of a sudden he fell to the ground and was lying still. Fritzie was called outside and tried to revive him, but it was too late. My grandfather suffered a heart attack and died under a tree at 83 years of age, helping a child get a toy. During his long life, he was always a kind, hardworking and happy man. The rest of the summer was very sad for us. The only thing that helped ease our sorrow a bit was the comfort of knowing that Pop got to live with us during that Catskill summer, where we were able to spend some great quality time together and he got to know and adore his little great-grandson before he passed. My mother gave me $1000 that Pop had given her to give to me. It was everything he had and he wanted me to have it. I felt and still feel special. Although it wasn't much money, he left me an inheritance of everlasting love.

But overall, the Catskills was a great experience for us, and when the season ended we closed the salon, counted our money, split the leftover supplies and journeyed south once again. Of course Fritzie and I first headed to Brooklyn to see the family, but not before stopping long enough to buy our first brand new car, a 1959 Ford Galaxy 500. How proud we were to start the drive back to Brooklyn with our success showing. I found that became a routine practice for the rest of our lives. Show your success so everyone would know that you're doing great was something I learned in Brooklyn as a child growing up; success begets success. There's nothing wrong with rewarding yourself after doing a great job, but only if you can truly afford it and if your accomplishments are real (and of course, don't forget to put 10% away for tomorrow). We returned to our apartment in Southwest Miami, I went back to work at the Fontainebleau Hotel and before we knew it, we had another son.

Little red-headed Larry Levine was our newest reason to give thanks, and in fact, he was born on Thanksgiving Day, 1959. We hadn't aimed for the holiday, but loved the timing. Larry was a beautiful seven and a half pound cherub with a smile that, from day one, would melt your heart. Everyone was happy for us and we felt blessed. Now we also needed a two-bedroom apartment, which luckily became available within the same building, so we moved upstairs and enjoyed the time together as a family.

The winter season was as good if not better than the previous year. I got more than my share of referrals and customers who became like family to me. But at 22, patience was not my strong suit, and time seemed to go very slowly for me. It usually does when you're waiting for something to happen. Around that time, I had a fortuitous meeting with a very kind woman named Molly Chesler. Meeting marvelous Molly Chesler started just about every good thing that happened to me from that point on and I'll always be thankful for the opportunity to become friends with her.

She lived in Toronto and New York, but we struck up a friendship while I was doing her hair in Miami. She sent in her daughter Ronnie, who was dating a nineteen-year old kid from Miami Beach by the name of Mel Harris (who would eventually become Ronnie's husband). Mel was a friendly, smart, handsome and industrious fellow, who was attending Miami University and seemed like a real "man on the move." While in college, he started a business selling madras shirts and jackets that made a lot of money. In fact, the trend spread across the country. Mel and I became fast friends, and in the years to come he will enter into my life many times to help me out in innumerable ways, and become like a brother to me.

Then one winter day Countess Marcella Borghese came into the salon. She was a lovely lady who was also very beautiful. I did her hair and she was extremely pleased, saying that it was an outstanding style for her. She must have seen something she liked in me, as she sent in Jerry Levitan, a Vice-President of Revlon to visit a few weeks later. Borghese was a protégé of Charles Revson, the founder of Revlon. I had heard that Revson helped her create her cosmetics line and later bought it as a subsidiary of the company. Jerry took me out to lunch and asked if I would be interested in relocating to Atlanta, GA to become a beauty expert and make-up artist for the company. I thought that it was a very exciting offer. I knew that I knew hair, but I also realized that knowing make-up would further expand my experience and undoubtedly help my career. So we agreed that after the winter season, I would go to New York and train as an expert on teaching women how to apply and wear a new product.

I was being asked to be one of seven people (the lucky seven, we liked to say) to present to the world a completely new make-up line that would revolutionize the cosmetics business. Charles Revson, one of the best merchandisers in the world, was preparing for the launch of Ultima Make-Up. This wasn't going to be the standard matching of lips and fingertips. The vision was to have an entire color selection that would change the whole concept of make-up forever, and I was going to be a part of it. Very exciting. Plus this meant I would get the chance to be trained by the best of the best – Mr. Pierre of Paris. I thought it was a great opportunity and jumped at it. Fritzie and I were excited about the prospect of working for one of the premiere companies in the world at the time and we started to envision our future.

During that time at the Fountainbleau, I met and worked for more celebrities and continued to grow my clientele and reputation, which included the likes of singers Jane Morgan (a great lady), Eydie Gorme (a sweetheart) and Connie Francis (the great singer and star). There were so many other wonderful people I had the pleasure to know, such as Mary Livingston, Jack Benny's wife. By the way, his act of being cheap and not spending money wasn't even close. In fact, the opposite was true. He regularly doled out $20 tips, which back then was huge. Along with being witty, Jack was also very charitable and kind.

I also learned that privacy was the utmost priority for those in the entertainment world. I recall watching Red Skelton sitting in the Fontainebleau Coffee Shop trying to eat lunch with his family. He kept getting interrupted for autographs, and he never refused. After almost one hour of not being able to eat (the line of people kept growing), his wife finally suggested they go upstairs and eat in their room. I saw Red another time, exiting a limousine with his wife while I was waiting for my car. He spotted a young girl, maybe eight or nine years old, standing with her mom. They looked at him with excitement and adulation. Then Red walked over to the girl and fell to his knees, hugging her and sobbing intensely. His wife pried him loose and helped him compose himself. The girl must have reminded him of his beloved daughter who had recently passed away from leukemia. That moment really affected me, and made me more inclined to act with compassion and kindness. You can never really tell the pain and loss that others are suffering, even when it may seem that they 'have it all' or are 'on top of the world.' I also thought about how there are so many ways you can make life happier for other people. Something as small as a hug can make all the difference in someone's day — or life, for that matter.

The season dwindled and the time to leave for New York came upon us. Revlon paid the rent on our apartment in Miami, as we didn't know exactly where we would be based after my training ended. We stayed in Brooklyn at my parents' apartment while I went to school to learn to be a beauty expert. Every day I arrived at 666 Fifth Avenue and went to our floor. There were seven of us from all over the country. Our instructor was Mr. Pierre from Paris, and our boss was Naomi Manners, a company Vice-President. In class we covered it all — application, packaging, branding and sales techniques. We tried to prepare for all of the questions a potential customer could have and have all the right answers at the ready.

> **Mini-Lesson:** *Learn something you didn't know the day before. To get something you never had, you have to do something you never did.*

The training also included closed-door classes in make-up application — on each other! What a riot. As well as personal application, the theory was that in order to be able to teach someone how, you have to truly know and understand the subject's experience. For the first month, it was very comical. Seeing yourself painted as a clown doesn't allow you to take yourself too seriously. However, by the second, third, and fourth months, it became very intense. One afternoon I got off the elevator to see Jerry Levitan about where I would ultimately be based, and I ran into Charles Revson himself. Mr. Revson saw me and said, "What are you doing wearing a sweater to work?" I was wearing a tie and a beautiful button down shirt and sweater that Fritzie had given me for my birthday. However, the official dress code for Revlon was dark tie, dark jacket and dark pants (or a black suit) and a white shirt. I quickly answered that my jacket was in the cleaners. He gave me an icy stare and told me in no uncertain terms to go home and get another jacket. "Are you kidding?" I asked. It was about 3 pm, and he was telling me at that hour to go home, change clothes and return.

He was serious. I told him I lived in Brooklyn and it would take an hour to go and another hour to come back. It would probably be after 5:30 p.m. before I made it back. He said, "Go now or never come back." So I swallowed my tongue (and my pride), got on the subway to Brooklyn, changed clothes, turned around and came back. When I finally did meet with Jerry much later that same day, he simply shrugged his shoulders and said, "Sorry kid, you just ran into the wrong guy on the wrong day." Live and learn, I guess. I never forgot the lesson that you have to dress for success if you want people to respect you. Perception is reality and people can only see what you present to them. Don't give them a reason to send you home.

> **Mini-Lesson:** *When you don't run the place, dress and behave the way you are told with a smile and the right attitude if you want to excel. His game, his rules.*

The good news was that we were nearing the completion of our training, and I was really starting to feel like an expert – ready to go out and teach the world. When I finally got my assignment, I was thrilled to find out that we would be going back to Miami. We still had our apartment, and although they weren't sure if I'd be based in Atlanta at some point later on, for now we got to live near some of the good friends we'd made. So back in Miami the Ultima product was already in department stores, but my job was to create in-store crowds by doing one or two small changes on a woman's face while instructing her how to do it herself. So I began travelling from store to store with a pop-up make-up bar and two mirrors that rose from inside. I started at Burdine's Department Store in Miami.

I also did product demonstrations for countless groups of women including the Legal Stenographers Association, the American Cancer Society, various sororities and a multitude of religious and charitable organizations. I enjoyed the work thoroughly and even got to make over Miss Universe pageant contestants at Burdine's. Boy was it fun. At the tender age of 23, I was speaking in front of large groups of people and doing well at it. Not only was it a great experience, but I realized that I really did love center stage. Sales increased dramatically, and I kept waiting for the applause from the home office in New York. All they'd say was that I was doing a good job, sales were great and to "keep up the good work." To my disappointment, no additional compensation was offered, but I just kept selling until I decided to leave the company and ask Buddy Maurice for my job back. Turns out I did not enjoy working for a large company with little communication and compensation not based on performance.

Around that time, a friend of mine who I met in the business, Sol Forster, invented a compact makeup refill ejector as there just wasn't a good way to change a refill in a beautiful compact without scratching the back of it. The metal ejector he invented did not scratch or even touch the outside. I thought it was genius. With Sol's approval, I sent the idea to Jerry Levitan, a VP at the home office who thought it was a great idea. Jerry assured me that he'd turn it over to the right people, and I was sure Revlon would buy it from my friend. I was so happy for Sol and expecting a nice bonus for bringing Sol's invention to the Revlon executives. How naïve I was. Soon after, I received a letter back from the legal department saying Revlon already had something similar to Sol's, but in plastic. I called the main office and asked to see it, but they said it was not ready for distribution, but no one within Revlon that I talked to had ever seen or heard of it, including Mr. Pierre.

About five months later, a plastic "thingamabob" came out to give out to customers who bought Revlon compacts. Although I never believed that it existed until they saw Sol's version, I couldn't prove it, but I did learn a hard lesson about protecting my ideas and documenting them properly. At that point, my regard for Revlon was decreasing fast and it would only get worse. Around the same time I was having a problem with a cyst on my back that needed to be operated on, so I went to the hospital. Although I had insurance through Revlon, they refused to pay me my salary while I was out sick. That was the last straw. We started talking about ending our contract arrangement but their opinion on how it should end differed drastically from mine. They wanted to prevent me from working as a beauty expert or hair stylist in the continental United States. I thought it was absurd for them to try to prevent me from supporting my family, and was ready for a fight.

A friend of mine named Harvey Steinberg was an Assistant District Attorney in Miami at the time and after I explained my situation he agreed to take on the giant. Revlon came down to Miami with three lawyers to fight me. Boy did I feel important. But I stood my ground. And when we went before the judge, it was decided that they would have to pay me for the time I was sick, and let me out of my contract. Although I was prevented from working in Dade County in the make-up industry for a number of months, I was allowed to practice hairstyling since I was a known hairstylist prior to working for them. I thought it was a very fair decision.

1960 - Miami, Florida

Once again, it was back to Buddy Maurice and the Fontainebleau Hotel. A new season was in full swing and I settled right in. Then to my surprise, Buddy asked me how I felt about going to New Orleans for a week to work at the Gus Mayers Department Store on Canal Street and promote his make-up, since I was now "the expert" he would say, to which we would both laugh. I had never been to New Orleans before, so naturally, I jumped at the chance to go. I took off with my Buddy Maurice makeup kit to the marvelous city of New Orleans. What a fantastic experience it was. The incomparable Louisiana accent, the Cajun and Creole food and the hospitality of the bayou — I loved it. I would end up listening to Al Hirt every night at the Al Hirt Saloon on Bourbon Street. The man had magic in his trumpet. I was grateful to be able to experience the great food, the amazing music, Bourbon Street — all of it.

The store had arranged for me to be a guest on the Terry Fletcher mid-day show the following morning. This was another first for me — being on a real live television show. The show's producers told me to get a blue shirt because the color blue showed up as white on black-and-white televisions. I did as instructed and bought one. Incidentally, Buddy later told me that he wouldn't pay for it. Anyway, the producers also told me that I wouldn't need to bring a model because women in the live audience would volunteer. That sounded fine to me. I was used to having people come in off the street and into my chair all the time, so why not here?

The day of the show I arrived on set extremely excited. The cameras started rolling and I was introduced as a former expert from Revlon. I got a warm reception from the audience. I looked into the crowd and asked if anyone wanted to come on stage and be my model. Although I couldn't see past the second row because of the lights, someone shouted out that there was a group in the audience from the Daughters of the American Revolution. I heard the word "daughters" so I automatically assumed they would be young, and I said, "Sure, come on up." A little old lady about 85 years old made her way up to the stage and I just about fell over. She came up and couldn't have been sweeter (although her skin couldn't have been more wrinkled). I had no choice but to think on my feet at that moment. My hairstyling background kicked in and I calmly took four hair clips out of my bag, pulled her hair back away from her face and fastened them tightly to her head. She immediately looked about twenty-five years younger. I then proceeded to apply Buddy Maurice's makeup on her, and wow, she looked a lot better. When I returned to Miami and the salon I came back to a hero's welcome. I found out that we were completely sold out of the Buddy Maurice product. They even hung a big sign at my station that read, "Welcome Home M. Walter, Our Hero." I felt like a million bucks. I basked in my success for the next few months.

> **Mini-Lesson:** *One of the most important skills is to think on your feet. The key is to believe in yourself — if you are confident that you will make the most out of any situation, you will.*

 Not long after, Buddy even offered me the opportunity to invest in his cosmetics company. I finally got up the nerve to ask Fritzie's Aunt Marie to loan me the money to buy in, but she said no. I never asked her for anything again, and although I accepted her decision with disappointment, it also prompted an inner resolve to make it on my own. I saw that there was really no other way. I told Buddy, "Thanks for the offer, but right now I have to say no." I was flattered that he offered me the opportunity to go into business with him and hoped that I'd be able to join him in a future venture, but just having the opportunity presented to me gave me a boost of confidence. I realized that it was only a matter of time until I would be in Buddy's position with the chance to help build something.

Around that time, the kind Mrs. Molly Chesler came back into my chair and my life, and through her, I reconnected with Mel Harris. I didn't realize how this would take my life in an entirely different direction. Mel was now married to Ronnie, Molly's daughter, and he was working for his father in law, Lou. Mel kindly invited me to a dinner that was sponsored by Dictograph Security Systems, a fire and burglar alarm company owned by Herman Perl, one of their business partners.

The dinner was at The Fontainebleau hotel and the room was filled with what felt like thousands of people in tuxedos and gowns. Many were holding signs that said "Herman Perl for President," and amazing prizes were being awarded, including fur coats, sterling silver tea sets, and even $10,000 cash. My eyes lit up like candles as I took it all in, incredulous. What an experience. Mel said to me, "One day, you'll be a part of all of this," to which I excitedly answered, "Sure!" But honestly, at that time I was unable to grasp the true scope of what I was being exposed to, nor the hard work needed to be part of it — yet. But my time was coming.

Then sometime in April, near the end of the season, Mel Harris sent another partner of his in to see me. His name was Marvin Hodes and he owned a chain of four beauty salons in the New York area, all called Marvin's. He said that he had heard a lot about me from Mel and Herman, and that they wanted me to manage a new salon they were building in the Catskills at the Concord Hotel, and while it was being built, he wanted me to work at his salon in Great Neck, Long Island. I was flattered and excited. So I took the offer home to think about and discuss with my partner, Fritzie, and after much discussion, we decided to make the move for our future. We said "goodbye for now" to all of our friends in Miami. Buddy had a goodbye party for us and graciously told me, "The door is always open." I said thanks to my mentor, and off we went back to New York and on to the next phase of our lives.

> **Mini-Lesson:** *I can't even begin to explain how great it is to have someone in your life who respects you enough and wants you to succeed so much that they will let you go, and if you don't succeed, you are welcome back home to the same wonderful job you had before you left. Of course you need to earn it, by having the right attitude, being enthusiastic and working to build relationships. Thank you, Buddy Maurice. I'll always be grateful for your generous spirit and willingness to help.*

1962 - Great Neck, NY

So I went to work in Great Neck, Long Island. It was a very wealthy community about thirty minutes from Manhattan. Marvin's Hairstyles was right in the center of town. Since I was now strictly known as Walter, this time around, there was no confusion regarding my name. Fritzie and I got an apartment in Fresh Meadows, Queens, and I did the reverse commute, against city-bound traffic, which made for a pleasant drive to work. Our good friend, Molly Chesler, lived in the Kings Point section of Great Neck, and with her referrals and my hard work, both my clientele and reputation grew.

It wasn't long before I built up a "good book" from Tuesday to Saturday and did anywhere from fifteen to twenty people a day, all the while building strong relationships with my customers and fellow stylists. The rapport I built with them helped me both personally and professionally. I was flattered to be invited to the homes of my clients — and what homes they had. Great Neck estates were big, beautiful and lavishly decorated. I had never been exposed to this type of wealth in a community before and I had an intense desire to find out how these people achieved this kind of life and level of success. This desire grew every day. So I asked a lot of questions and did a lot of listening.

One day, an especially nice client of mine named Mrs. Shirley Kleinman invited me to her home to have dinner with her and her family. Her husband Sy Kleinman was a senior partner at Golenbock & Barell, a high profile New York City law firm. He was also one of the funniest men I have ever met. A collector of religious artifacts and a very interesting man in general, he shared his home, his food, his family and his ideals with me generously and with great humor. During our meal I got up the nerve to ask him the all-important question: "How?" "How did you do it? How did you achieve all this?" Sy looked at me seriously and said, "The only person standing in the way of your success is you. If you truly want it, the option is entirely yours." I countered with, "Sure, you can say that because your family helped you to get a good education, but how in the world does someone like me make it to that level?" He replied, "Well, how badly do you want success? How high do you want to go? What price are you willing to pay?" Although I found it difficult to process at the time, I took those questions to heart, and in fact, they are still with me today. And I pose them to others all the time, including my children and grandchildren. When I think back to that dinner, I believe those words opened a little door in my mind — a door that promised the start of something new and something big. Something that I had instinctively always known, but was never able to fully articulate and embrace. I began to believe that it really was all up to me and how far I wanted to go — it always had been and it still is today.

After that dinner, I continued to ask questions of successful people and really listen to their answers. I found that most were truly willing to share their stories of success. A gentleman by the name of Joe Schwartz, whose wife, Ruth, was another client of mine, was also very generous with his advice and life experience. Joe was in the oil business, and I mean a whale of an oil business. In fact, the names of his companies were Whale Oil and Paragon Oil. He owned the largest group of holding tanks in the New York City area for the Amoco Corporation. Joe helped me to see that the real business I was in was not hair styling, but the business of building "relationships." That was a real eye-opener for me. "Imagine the possibilities," I thought.

And with this newest realization, I recognized the need to further my education, because if anyone was going to take me seriously in business, I would have to know something about the business world. So I sent away for a home study course through the Alexander Hamilton Institute. It may not have been the Ivy League, but it was the best I had available to me at the time, and I made the most that I possibly could out of it. I studied all the time – while waiting for clients to come into the salon, during lunch, during dinner and even late at night. The concepts finally started to come together for me after about eight or nine months. But that was only part of it. I would also have to become comfortable with this new image of myself—that of as a businessman asking the almighty question, "How Can I Help You?" other than in the hair and makeup world.

Well, the one thing that I never lacked was confidence, and soon after, I had what I thought was a great idea. I would ask Molly Chesler if she thought I had what it would take to be an assistant to her husband, Lou.

She thought for a moment and replied, "Why not!?!" So Molly arranged for an appointment for me to meet with him at their home. Although I knew Molly for some time and was great friends with her daughter and son in law Mel, I had never been to her home or met her husband. I had only heard about him and what an imposing figure he was — both physically and with regard to the level of success he had achieved.

The following Monday, I knocked on the door of one the largest houses I had ever seen in my life. I had seen mansions in the movies, but none of them even compared to this. The feeling I had in the pit of my stomach let me know this is what dreams are made of. I was dressed in the best suit and tie I owned and my shoes were newly shined. I had prepared what I was going to say at the meeting, and didn't doubt even for a moment that he would say yes to my proposal. I would become his personal assistant. A dream job that would allow me entrée into a whole new way of life and to all of the finer things that went along with it. Talk about naïve.

I stood at the front door of the mansion but couldn't find the doorbell, so I started knocking on the door. I knocked for about five minutes, until my hands hurt. I started to think that no one was home when finally, the butler answered. He looked at me quizzically and asked why I didn't just ring the bell. He pointed to the center of the door, and I felt very stupid. I told him that I had an appointment with Mr. Chesler and gave him my name. He told me to come in and wait in the room on the right. He'd be right back.

The front hallway was twice the size of my entire apartment with an incredible view of the Long Island Sound. I found the small waiting room on the right with a settee and a mirror opposite it. I sat down and waited for what seemed like forever. A few weeks prior, Fritzie and I were invited as guests of Molly to the world movie premiere of "West Side Story" one of the movies Lou produced. I started thinking about all of the varied and successful businesses that Mr. Chesler owned: Seven Art Films, Mirrisch Films, General Development Corporation, American Totalizator Corporation. He was even a founding partner of the Grand

Bahamas Island Development Company on the island of Freeport. As I sat there thinking and dreaming, I caught myself in the mirror and began to laugh, as I looked like a Little Boy Blue painting.

Disturbing my pleasant thoughts, in walked Lou Chesler, a giant of a man about 300 pounds and 6'4" tall. Following close behind was this tiny man, who made Lou seem even larger. He stopped where I was sitting and said, "What the hell are you sitting in the powder room for? You fags don't know nothing. C'mon, follow me." "Where do I go from here?" I thought. About ten feet down the hall was his den (the room the butler was actually referring to and where I was supposed to be waiting). It had several big black couches and club chairs, was lined with bookshelves and had a bar, TV and a huge desk in front of an enormous picture window.

At that moment, I felt two feet tall. I thought that I blew it and that there was no way I could dig out of the deep hole I had just created for myself. Lou introduced the small man with him as Eddie Arcaro. Then Mr. Chesler said, "What the hell are you here for? What do you want?" I had almost forgotten what I was there for. I felt very nervous and rocked to my very foundation. I managed to stammer, "I'd like a job as your assistant." They looked at each and started laughing. Mr. Chesler said, "Well, then what the hell am I supposed to do with Arcaro, here? He's my public relations director and my assistant." "Are you kidding?" he asked, stunned. So much for my brilliant plan. I apologized and told them I didn't know that he had an assistant. They began talking amongst themselves as if I wasn't even there. I stood there in shock and didn't move for a few minutes, which seemed like hours. I felt completely invisible, but tried to remain calm and seem unruffled.

Then, in walked Mel Harris and Alan Chesler, Lou's son. I was so happy to see them! It was like being thrown a life-preserver in the middle of the ocean. We said hello and I shook hands heartily. Mel asked me if I wanted to join them all at Aqueduct Race Track. Looking for a way out of the current situation and a chance to redeem myself, I quickly agreed. So I followed them out the front door to an awaiting limousine and chauffeur. The four of them got in the rear and asked if I wouldn't mind riding in the front seat next to the driver. I thought that was special, so I happily agreed (what a moron I was). I didn't say much during the ride aside from thanking them for taking me along.

As we headed to Lou's private box at Aqueduct, I listened to them talk about his horse, "Away with You," who was running in the sixth race. Eddie said there wasn't another horse in this race and that we had to win. As they talked, it became clear to me that Eddie Arcaro was actually the most successful and well-known jockey in the world. I was very impressed. When we got to the track they all headed to the window and bet big bucks. Chesler bet thousands and Arcaro, Mel and Alan bet hundreds of dollars. Who was I to question? I had about $60 in my pocket, and not wanting to go against the guys, I bet it all on "Away With You." I was a moron.

While I was reading the program I spotted the name of a jockey, Walter Blum. I knew him. He was my old friend, Little Walter, who I grew up with in Brooklyn. At 4'11" and 96 pounds, with size 4 feet, he was a perfect candidate for jockey-hood, and he apparently pursued his calling. I recalled a Jewish holiday back when we were kids. All the neighborhood boys travelled to the Belmont race track to watch Walter ride as an apprentice on a horse called Hatikva (which means "hope" in Hebrew). We cheered him on and he won. Boy, did we celebrate. Walter moved out of Brooklyn and we lost contact, but seeing his name was on the program filled me with pride and excitement.

We still had two races until the sixth race, so I excused myself and headed down toward the Jockey Room. I was stopped by security and told them that my friend, the jockey Walter Blum, wanted to see me. They didn't believe me, but they did agree to take a message back to Walter for me. Walter immediately came out and we hugged and talked for a few minutes. Then he went back to dressing and I went back to Mr. Chesler's box. It was finally time for the sixth race, and as luck would have it, "Away with You" basically ran away with our money. We all lost, big time. And guess who won? That's right, Little Walter from Brooklyn, and because it was a long shot, it paid big time. I couldn't believe it. I didn't even have the decency or smarts to bet $2 on my childhood friend. How stupid I was, I thought. But it got even worse.

The guys said they were now heading to New York City for a meeting and then dinner. Everyone said goodbye to me and left. I then understood what a poor dejected loser feels like. Needless to say, with my car stranded in Kings Point, Great Neck and me totally broke with no money, I started walking home. During the next four hours, I kept asking myself how I allowed this to happen. Was I crazy? What was I thinking? What a fool. I didn't belong in this world. I walked and walked and thought of everything a father of two small children, who just lost all the extra money the family needed for the next two weeks, would say to himself.

> **Mini-Lesson:** *Never bet the farm if you don't really believe in something. There comes a time in your life when you realize who matters and who never did. Try harder to do the right thing for the right reasons rather than trying to impress people.*

Then I started to think about how I was going to explain this to Fritzie. When I finally got home, I ashamedly told her that I blew it. Of course, she had no idea what I was talking about, so I took her through the full story of the day. When I was finished getting the day's events and mishaps off my chest to my wife, she was as understanding as ever and I felt a lot better. Overall, life was still good, and I was happy to be back in New York with my family. Even though I was beginning to envision the life I could have for myself and my family, there was still a lot of hard work to do.

Life Lesson #5 - How High Do You Want to Go? It's Up to You:

The more I was exposed to successful people and opened myself up to how they thought, the more I realized that even though we may have come from different worlds and upbringings, there was really no good reason that I could not achieve what they could — other than my own excuses.

The kind (and blunt) English lady who told me, point blank that my diction needed help, did me a huge favor. Although I never got a chance to properly thank her (and I'm frankly, not sure I would've at the time), her honesty was like cold water in my face. Hard to take, but something I needed to experience. I'm glad that I was open to her feedback. Often times, moving forward means shedding an old skin (and sometimes even changing your name).

Along the same lines, when I had that dinner with Sy and he said *"The only person standing in the way of your success is you. If you truly want it, the option is entirely yours,"* I didn't understand at the time how true that statement was, but he couldn't have been more right. If you're really serious about making the most out of every opportunity presented to you, you need to be prepared to do whatever it takes.

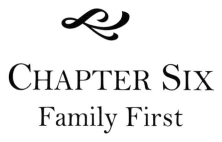

CHAPTER SIX
Family First

LIFE LESSON #6...
WHEN OPPORTUNITY KNOCKS,
ANSWER THE DOOR

"Your children are not your children.
They are the sons and daughters of Life's longing for itself."
— Kahlil Gibran

ritzie was pregnant again and I'm happy to say that she went through the next nine months very well. Everyone at the salon was hoping we would have a healthy girl. I remember her delivery day so clearly. I took Steve and Larry to my Mom and Dad's apartment in Brooklyn, and then I took Fritzie to Long Island Jewish Hospital. I waited for nine hours when the obstetrician finally came out and told me to go home and rest. I drove to Brooklyn, arriving at approximately 8:30pm. As I sat down to eat dinner, the phone rang. When I answered, the doctor said, "Congratulations!" I asked him anxiously, "Boy or girl?" His reply was, "Girl." I smiled and shouted to Mom that we had a girl, and with that the doctor said, "You didn't let me finish…" I asked, "Is she alright?" He said "She's fine, but…" "But what?" I was so nervous. No one says "but" unless there's a problem. He continued to explain that Fritzie gave birth to two identical twin girls. Well, you could have knocked me over with a feather. I couldn't even speak.

I recall my mother putting a wet towel on the back of my neck and asking me what was wrong. I said, "Mom, you're not going to believe this, but we've got twin girls!" She screamed so loudly with joy that I thought she would blow a gasket. She kept hugging me and the boys. I jumped in the car and drove to the hospital at about eighty miles per hour, hoping a cop would stop me just so I could tell somebody how excited I was to have twin girls.

When I got to the hospital and saw Fritzie, we hugged and laughed and she told me that I was nuts for shouting all over the maternity wing of the hospital. We were so very happy. Leslie and Lori Levine's arrival was one blessed day. Our family was complete. Thank God. I made a few calls late that night and when I went to work at Marvin's Salon the next day, I arrived to see a huge sign reflected on all of the mirrored walls that read: "It's Twin Girls For The M. Walter Levine Family!" I passed out cigars to women and men alike and was congratulated like I had won the Nobel Peace Prize. To my great surprise the next day the news spread and my customers and friends began sending presents — two of everything. We even got two high chairs from Saks Fifth Avenue. I couldn't believe it. The kind people of Great Neck were so generous, it seemed we wouldn't need to buy anything for the twins until they were two years old.

> **Mini-Lesson:** *Treat people the way you want to be treated — it was obviously the motto of the wonderful people of Great Neck. They were more than kind to Fritzie and I, as well as our growing family.*

Our family was expanding and we needed a bigger apartment. We moved to a two bedroom, one bath place in Fresh Meadows, across the street from the movie theater. Steve and Larry had one bedroom, Fritzie and I had the other with our new twins, Leslie and Lori, sharing a crib. We folded a sheet to divide the crib length-wise, enabling us to have Leslie on one side and Lori on the other. When one baby woke crying, we'd change or feed her, but before long the other twin would wind up waking. It became a juggling act, and we had very little sleep for a few months. The reality and costs of having four children was starting to set in. Our lives would never be the same, but it was worth every penny. Getting and giving that much love is quite a feeling. But I did need to work harder in order to make ends meet. I convinced Marvin to let me work longer hours and keep the salon open later so I could take in more clients.

One day at the salon, one of my customers suggested that I consider opening up my own salon. I mentioned that the people who brought me from the Fontainebleau Hotel in Miami Beach were planning to set me up in a new salon at the Concord Hotel in the Catskills, that I would manage and also receive a percentage of sales. My customer reminded me that nothing promised is assured and strongly encouraged me to meet with some friends of her husband who she said might be interested in backing me in my own salon. I figured that I had nothing to lose, plus her belief in me was rather flattering, so I agreed to a meeting. I met the two gentlemen for dinner in Great Neck and we discussed the idea of a partnership whereby they would invest in a new salon for me, and the profits would be split 50/50. I had mentioned the meeting coming up to an attorney friend named Mike Fox whose wife was also a client of mine. Mike made me promise to call him before I agreed to anything. After dinner, they pulled a suitcase full of money out from under the table, and said that they wanted to invest. I was thrilled and honored. I felt incredible to have this offer — how fantastic.

The men agreed to my request to make a quick phone call to my attorney friend to discuss the offer. They handed me the suitcase and I made the call to Mike, elated by my good fortune. After Mike listened to the offer they had made me, he told me to have them put it in writing for him to review. He also asked me what collateral the men had asked for. I asked Mike to hold on. I put the phone down and walked back over to the men to share my friend's recommendations and questions. Their reply was, "We don't need no contract. And we don't need no collateral either. We've got you." I returned to the phone and repeated to Mike what they had said. I'll never forget Mike's next words to me. He said, "Put down that suitcase, and get the hell out of that restaurant now!" I did exactly as he said and never looked back. I'll always be grateful to Mike and his very astute legal advice that day. I wanted my own business, but not that badly.

Mini-Lesson: *He who laughs last...lives.*

Luckily, the balance of my time working and living on Long Island was relatively uneventful. I worked long, hard hours, continuing my self-directed business studies and then finally, the salon at the Concord Hotel was ready to be opened for business. As promised, Mel Harris asked me to manage it, and in addition to my salary, I was also given a small piece of the business as part of my compensation. Now I would learn directly from the pros how to run a business and how to truly harness the power of incentive.

1962 - The Concord Hotel, Catskill Mountains, NY

After wonderful goodbyes and promises to keep in touch with the co-workers and clients who had become my friends "working family," we departed to Monticello, high in the Catskill Mountains of New York. We were able to buy our first house — a split-level with a one-car garage that cost $19,000, a ton of money to us back then. We decorated the house in the "Early American" style and we were so proud of it. I took to the new job and responsibilities like a duck to water. The Concord Hotel was one of the largest and most famous hotels in America at the time. It had 1800 rooms, three large kitchens and a dining room that could feed 3500 people in one sitting. It also had a very wealthy clientele that didn't mind spending money for the things they wanted. Irving Cohen was the maître'd and ran the place like an army general. Everything and everyone had to be perfect.

> **Mini-Lesson:** *When given the chance to learn from the pros, you need to listen, practice and grow. Be proud to be part of a great opportunity, and don't be afraid to bring your own positive energy to it — help to grow the business.*

Lucky for me, Irving took me under his wing when I arrived at the Concord, which helped ease my transition. He introduced me to everyone and showed me how things really worked at the hotel. He even told me that anytime I wanted to eat, I could just come up to the dining room and be taken care of, which was a huge compliment. Although I only took him up on it once or twice, it was a very thoughtful gesture on his part. One night Irving even took me to a Masonic Lodge meeting nearby, where he was a member. I learned that every President of the United States, except John F. Kennedy, was a mason — even George Washington. At Irving's urging, I became one too.

I also became fast friends with Arthur Winarick, the owner of The Concord. We had a lot in common. He was an immigrant from Russia (like my father) and a former barber (like me) on New York's Lower

East Side. Since we practiced the same trade, I asked Arthur how a barber got the money to build something as magnificent as the Concord Hotel. He seemed to like my curiosity and passion for life and enjoyed spending time hanging out with us in the beauty salon. He thought we'd done a terrific job fixing it up and he was very happy with the swift business we were doing, handling his guests with the respect he was hoping for.

Sometimes I'd join Arthur for tea or lemonade at Mrs. Jay's Dining Room and he would tell me great stories of his life. How he came to this country penniless and wound up the barber for a gang called Murder Incorporated, on the Lower East side of New York City. He would cut their hair and give them shaves, then one day during Prohibition they told him he would be going into the hair tonic business. Since hair tonic needed alcohol, it was a great cover for them, and just like that Jeris Hair Tonic was started. By the time Prohibition ended, Arthur had made enough money to buy a small 29-room hotel with a nice porch in Kiamesha Lake called Mrs. Jay's Bungalow Colony. He continued to expand and expand until it eventually became The Concord Hotel — one of the greatest hotels in the United States.

Although the Concord crowd was considered seasonal, the hotel was busy most of the year. It had two great golf courses and also catered to skiers during the winter. It was a wonderful year-round resort. I had a great staff of 29 and business got better every day. Even some owners and customers from competing hotels, such as Grossinger's (which was the inspiration for the fictitious Kellerman's Mountain Resort featured in the film Dirty Dancing) came to our salon to get their hair done. But they would never use their real names when making an appointment for fear of being found out.

Many of the entertainers that I had gotten to know at the Fontainebleau Hotel in Miami came to perform at the Concord during the summer months. Connie Francis, Jane Morgan, Sammy Davis, Jr., Steve Lawrence & Eydie Gorme were just some of the acts that regularly appeared at the

Concord. Eydie and I really hit it off great. She even asked if I would come to Manhattan to do her hair whenever she was in town and I agreed. I had similar friendships and arrangements with Jane Morgan and other performers as well. The crazy and loveable Buddy Hackett came into the salon one time screaming at the top of the lungs and acting silly while his wife and mother were getting their hair done. Everyone couldn't help but crack up. It felt like one long, non-stop party.

One Saturday night in August, Sammy Davis Jr. was scheduled to appear. It also happened to be my Fritzie's birthday. That afternoon at around 1pm, the salon was humming with activity. I was standing at the desk near the front door and Sammy walked by. We looked at each other in recognition. He remembered that I had done his wife's hair down at the Fontainebleau and he came in to give me a hug. He asked if I was going to see his show that night. I told him that I certainly was, and that it was my wife's birthday so we had a party of ten people coming to the show to celebrate with us. He asked what my wife's name was and told me to bring her backstage after the show to say hello. When he walked away I was on "Cloud Nine." Not only had Arthur Winarick arranged for Fritzie and our guests to have a fabulous dinner at the hotel that night, now this. It was promising to be a wonderful evening. After dinner, Mr. Winarik had reserved the front table next to the stage for us and had two bottles of champagne and a birthday cake waiting. Fritzie was beaming. You couldn't have asked for a sweeter moment in life — only it got better.

They introduced Sammy and as the orchestra started playing, he walked on stage singing one of my favorite songs, "I've Gotta Be Me." The audience swelled in applause. He was great. But at the very end of the song, his voice cracked on the last note. He stopped the orchestra abruptly and told the audience that they came to hear his best and he wasn't pleased that his voice broke on the last note. If the audience wouldn't mind, he would like to start the song all over again. The audience indicated their approval and he sang the entire song again. This time it was perfect and at the end the crowd gave him a standing ovation. What a showman he was. He then asked if the audience would continue standing and if they wouldn't mind helping him sing "Happy Birthday" to a friend of his in the audience. He started and then a room full of 3500 people joined in to sing "Happy Birthday Dear Fritzie... Happy Birthday to You." Fritzie was red-faced as can be, but glowing. I know she felt very special that night, maybe more than any other time before in her life. Does life get any better than that? It's an amazing memory.

> **Mini-Lesson:** *Try to remember that although every journey has a destination, great stops can happen along the way when you create relationships. This was one memorable stop.*

Monticello is a small town, and in a very short period of time Fritzie and I came to know a large amount of people in the area. One day, a few friends called and asked if I would like to come to a meeting, as they were going to start a chapter of the Jaycee's in Monticello. The Jaycee's were an organization of young men under the age of thirty-five that would work for the betterment of the community and teach men how to organize, speak in front of a group and do community service. I said "Sure" and went along with them. About fifty men showed with an average age of about twenty-seven. I must have said something right during the meeting, because the next thing I knew, I was being elected President. There's no telling exactly what was said afterward, but from the anger of a few men in the room after the vote, I felt like I took away the ball and no one else could play. Oh well.

I thought that no one would show up for my first meeting, but boy, was I wrong. Many came and they brought many others. The charter group wound up having over eighty members. We did some wonderful things for the community and helped a lot of people that couldn't help themselves. Some of our accomplishments involved cleaning up the main street, planting flowers and helping to feed the poor by distributing food from local restaurants that would have been thrown away. There were many other worthwhile projects we spearheaded that raised money to help others in need.

I got to lead a terrific group of professionals – local merchants and business owners including lawyers, physicians and the leaders of tomorrow. We had a wonderful member by the name of Jack McBride, who was the Assistant District Attorney of Sullivan County. He wanted to enter politics and one day he got his opportunity. Assemblyman and House Minority Leader, Hyman Mintz died, and there was an election to fill his seat. Our group said we would help Jack get into the race for Mintz's seat. We did and he won. Jack's Dad helped tremendously as he owned McBride's Dairy and helped out financially and with contacts. My First Vice-President, an attorney named Leo Glass, also went to Albany with Jack. They believed they could make a difference. Unfortunately, things didn't go very well for them there.

When they tried to buck the "good ole boys" system that was long in place, the good ole boys weren't very happy about it, and promptly tried to get rid of them. It was soon decided to redistrict the area and roll Sullivan County up into a much larger district where the Assemblyman had been in office forever. We lost that battle, but I did learn a few things about politics and how hard it is to fight city hall. In any event, getting elected to the Jaycee's was a big thing in my life. During the year I was in office I met the governor of New York at the time, Nelson Rockefeller, at a luncheon. We had a conversation that I'll never forget. He said, "Walter, politics are all about money and power, and I have both. The trick is not to abuse either one." It was a lesson well learned, and the experience convinced me to stay out of politics.

> **Mini-Lesson:** *You have to have passion for what you do and love it for the right reasons. When you do, you are able to lead from trust, not fear, and put your energy into constructive actions.*

Business was terrific and my name and reputation grew. But what sometimes happens when everything seems to be going well, something comes out of nowhere and shakes you to your core. Larry was not doing all the things that little boys his age normally did and we were getting concerned. He was kind of hyper and he didn't speak or communicate. We thought there may have been something wrong, but we prayed that there wasn't. He was such a happy child. He was very sweet to Steve and the twins, always smiling and wanting to give love. He asked for nothing in return except Carvel or Dairy Queen ice cream and chocolate fudge.

Although Larry really didn't speak much at all, Steve could figure out what he wanted most of the time, so he had most of his needs met. But we started to become concerned, and decided to take him to see a doctor in Monticello who was recommended by one of my clients. After carefully examining Larry, he told us that he believed Larry definitely had a problem, and he used the word "retarded" when describing his condition. We went into shock. This couldn't be happening. By the way, although nowdays the word retarded may not be considered politically correct by some, back then it was the socially accepted term for the condition, and I still use it — not at all disrespectfully. I certainly know and respect the words "developmentally disabled."

The summer season had just ended. For a few days we tried to go on with our daily lives, but we realized that for the first time ever Fritzie and I really needed to get away. We had never left our children before, and in fact hadn't been on vacation alone since our honeymoon (if you could call that a vacation). Although we always chose to think positively, having four children and trying to earn enough to keep our heads above water was taking its toll, and this new problem with Larry laid very heavily on our minds and hearts. A friend mentioned a gambling junket to Las Vegas that she thought we should look into. Travel was free, but they hoped that you'd gamble enough to make up for your travel expenses many times over. Having limited resources we decided to try it. We arranged for my mom to come up from Brooklyn to take care of the children and Arthur Winarick promised he would stop by or send someone to see if there was anything they needed. We were so grateful for their help.

We made our way to the airport, and onto a non-stop private flight to Las Vegas on a "Big Julie" junket (trips arranged by the famous Julius

Weintraub "Big Julie" — who basically created the concept of the 'gambling junket' — they were big at that time). The pilot announced before take-off that, "a good time would be had by all." It was a happy crowd to say the least, and we were happy to join the party. The next time we heard from our pilot was when he announced that we would be stopping somewhere in Texas because we had run out of liquor and if everyone would chip in we could buy some more booze. We all laughed the rest of the way. Can you imagine? What we thought would be a seven-hour flight, took us twelve hours, but we arrived happy.

We were picked up and driven to our beautiful hotel, although our room was no larger than a walk-in closet. And considering we packed enough clothes for three weeks even though we were on a four day trip, things were pretty tight. But we had a great time and actually won a little bit of money gambling. I even learned how to shoot craps. It was a nice, well-needed vacation, and we talked about coming back again someday. We actually wound up going back many times, and Vegas became one of our favorite places to visit. Luckily, I had learned back at the racetrack to never bet the farm.

Then to our delight and surprise, we ran into Ali Harris, Mel Harris' father at one of the casinos, the Dunes Hotel located across the street from The Flamingo. He welcomed us heartily and asked if Mel knew we were there. We told him that it was an impulsive trip and that no one really knew about it. He arranged for us to have lunch at one of the lovely hotel restaurants, while he called his son who was now living in California. Mel called us back within minutes and we took the call right in the booth we were sitting at. They brought the phone to Ali Harris. Mel said he would fly to Vegas to meet us that evening to take us out for a fabulous dinner and a show at the Sands. We were so excited. Mel arrived in Vegas as planned and whisked us off to an amazing night on the town with him as our host. After the show he even introduced us to the girls from the chorus line, who I must say were absolutely gorgeous. It was a great evening that we thoroughly enjoyed. At the end of the night we told him about our problem with Larry, and his heart went out to us.

So much so that he said, "Forget about the junket. I'll arrange for you to go to California and enjoy the next four days in my house in Beverly Hills." He took care of the plane tickets and gave me the keys to his Cadillac convertible as well as his beautiful home. It was the first time we had ever been on the West Coast and as we drove around the Hills of Beverly, we couldn't believe that we were really there. We were greeted at Mel's house by a houseman who was expecting us and got us settled in. The house was like a dream - spacious, immaculate, lavishly decorated and with a breathtaking view. There was a swimming pool in back with a large dolphin fountain. At dusk, the lights that hung above all of the artwork throughout the house would turn on automatically. It was very impressive. Mel had obviously done very well for himself in California (and everywhere). I was so proud of him, and I still am today.

> **Mini-Lesson:** *Life is all about relationships. Mel gave a gift of more than money. He gave of himself for our benefit —a great lesson in integrity and emotion. Thank you, Mel. It really helped us to learn to give back.*

Across the street a huge candelabra sat on the lawn of one of Mel's neighbors. It turned out that his neighbor was none other than the talented and flamboyant pianist, Liberace. While we were there, two party invitations were hand-delivered for Mel — one from Elizabeth Taylor and the other from Harry Belafonte. I truly felt like we were in a dream, or at least on a movie set, as Mel had arranged for everything we could possibly imagine, including a private tour of Universal Studios and dinner at the finest restaurants in town. No one would accept our money because Mel had made all the calls personally. Mel arranged for us to have dinner at The Bistro restaurant, one of the best in town, and apparently quite a celebrity haunt. We were seated at the second table to the left of the door, a very good location the maitre'd informed us. The likes of Sal Mineo, Hugh O'Brien, Lana Turner, Red Button and other movie industry types kept parading by our table as they arrived.

Many of them surprisingly greeted me by name, saying "Hi, Walt" as they came in. I kept saying "Hi" back to them, even though I'd never met them. For a moment I thought that Mel might be playing a joke on me.

But then an older man sitting at the first table to the left of the door turned around to me and said, "You must be very important for all those people to say hello to you. Who are you?" I told him that I was Walter Levine, and that I was a hairstylist visiting from New York. He shook my hand and said, "Hello, I'm Walt Disney. I think those people were probably saying hello to me." I didn't recognize his face, but I certainly knew the name. Of course that's who everyone was saying hello to. At that moment I was so embarrassed I felt like Dumbo himself. As I blushed many shades, we all had a good laugh. Even though I was a legend in my own mind that day, Mr. Disney was gracious and wonderful. What a class act. We all laughed!

> **Mini-Lesson:** *Don't believe all of your own press notices. Have a sense of humor — I guarantee you'll need it one day.*

It was time to return home and back to reality. We knew it was up to us to take the bull by the horns and do everything we could to get Larry the help he needed. So we went to New York City and to see a line-up of specialists who told us to "Take him home and love him," or "Put him in an institution because there is nothing that could be done for him," and everything in between. We decided that we needed to follow our own hearts and instincts. Even though we didn't have much extra money we knew that this had to be a priority, so we decided to try to get someone to live in our home and help Fritzie with the kids while making sure that Larry had his needs met. Larry was still very dependent and needed a lot of help, including help to go to the bathroom. We went to an agency in New York City and we wound up hiring the first girl that we interviewed. Her name was Viola, and she fit right in with her sweet face, great attitude and a willingness to help all of our children, especially Larry. She was from the south and was grateful to be with us and away from the tough life she led back home.

Back at the Concord Salon, the numbers were peaking, my income was increasing and I was happy that I had a piece of the action. I had become good friends with a very lovely lady named Frenchie, who was in charge of Concord hotel reservations. Her husband also happened to be the talented and hilarious Marty Allen of the famous comedy team, Allen and Rossi. I would occasionally work on Marty's wigs for his shows — wild black hair — fun! At about 6:30 one Saturday evening, I received a call from Frenchie that she had the next greatest star since Judy Garland sitting in her office. She was going to appear and sing at the nine o'clock show and needed my help. I told her that I was on my way out and had plans for the evening, but she implored, "Walter, please do this for me."

> **Mini-Lesson:** *In order to get favors, you gotta give some. Don't forget, the business that you're in — that ultimately, we're all in: "The People Business."*

Hoping that if I hurried I could still pick up the pizza I had ordered from Carlo's Restaurant and make it home on time or just a little late for dinner with the family as planned, I reluctantly agreed and told Frenchie to send her in. "By the way," I asked, "What's her name?" "Barbra Streisand," Frenchie said. I had never heard of her. Within minutes, I felt a tap on the shoulder and turned around. I saw a young woman in torn sneakers, overalls with one side unhooked, a Brooklyn College sweatshirt and hair that definitely needed attention. "Hi! I'm Barbra," she chirped. I also saw a lovely face filled with determination, desire, real passion and a beautiful and unique nose. I said, "Hi, I'm Walter. Let's get your hair shampooed." A small and sweet woman named Ada Greenburg, who worked for me doing shampoos, manicures, and pedicures, took Barbra in back and washed her hair. Ada was Mel Harris' cousin and the mother of one of the fastest growing stars of the business world, Maurice (Hank) Greenberg, who would later found and run the AIG Insurance Company. Ada returned Barbra to my chair, where I trimmed and set her hair, then put her under the dryer.

When I finished, Barbra was very pleased and told me she'd never looked better. "Hello gaw-geous!" She asked if I would please be her guest at her performance that night. I thanked her for the offer but explained that I had plans for pizza with my family and wished her great luck. She said, "Bring the whole family." I decided to head home for pizza with the family. The next day at the salon, while I was cleaning up (since I didn't get a chance to the night before), about twenty people poked their heads in to ask if I went to Barbra's show. I was told over and over that she was a huge hit — just brilliant. Her talent amazed the crowd, and she received many standing ovations. I was also told that she mentioned my name a few times, and thanked me for doing her hair.

A few months later, the talented girl from Brooklyn went on to star in a wonderful show called Funny Girl, the life story of Fanny Brice, and the rest is history. Even though Fritzie and I have had the opportunity to see Barbra perform and visit with her backstage on several occasions since then, I wish I had accepted her kind offer, let the pizza go, grabbed the entire family and been her special guest at that show. Oh well, live and learn. In any event, it was an honor to be a part of her debut at the Concord Hotel, and it is a memory I will always treasure. One very positive outcome from that day was a great personal relationship and friendship with Barbra's manager, Marty Erlichman, his wife Miko and son JJ, who was also Bette Midler's manager.

One day, during a visit to New York, I decided to take a side trip to New Jersey and see Herman Perl. Herman was doing some very exciting things in the beauty business, and was preparing to take his company public. I told Herman that the Concord salon was doing very well and that I wanted to talk about the salon's future, as well as mine. I had some ideas about expanding and opening salons at other big hotels in the area. He told me that if I thought I could handle it, to go for it. Herman then asked me if I would be interested in running a small cosmetic company that he was thinking of buying, called Jon Pierre. I jumped at the chance and dove in wholeheartedly. In the next few months, I opened beauty salons at several hotels in the Catskills including The Brown's Hotel (which was Jerry Lewis' favorite place), and The Homawack Hotel, where we also offered the Jon Pierre line of cosmetics for sale.

Before long, I took over all aspects of the cosmetics company including manufacturing, shipping, advertising, training, and sales. I put together a sales force called the Jon Pierre Girls, who went door to door with small kits to sell product, similar to the Avon and Mary Kay ladies. We came out with a lipstick called Neutratone, which enabled the individual chemistry in each woman's body to be neutralized so that the color in the lipstick tube was the true color on their lips. We advertised in Vogue, Mademoiselle, Harpers and other magazines and the orders flowed in. We were even carried in some department stores, including Lord & Taylor. The growth was so amazing that we had to move the shipping from a small rented warehouse space in Monticello down to Herman Perl's large headquarters in New Jersey where Herman's father-in-law who ran Beauty Industries took over the shipping.

Although my professional life was flourishing, back at home Fritzie and I had our hands full with Larry. We found out about a Dr. Eugene Spitz at the Center for Human Potential in a place called Media, Pennsylvania, outside of Philadelphia, and made an appointment. With prayers and emotions riding high, we started the drive from Monticello at 5:30am. When we arrived at 8:30am, the line to get in was already 30 people deep. Dr. Spitz was a leader in his field, and apparently one of the nicest men in the world who didn't know how to say no to anyone who needed his help. He started his day at 6:30am and worked straight through till 6pm. What a great man. He even took patients during lunch, asking questions and making notes while eating. He also flew around the United States with a personal pilot to perform surgery. We met families from around the world at the center, including royalty. We all came to find help for the same problem.

Part of Dr. Spitz's program was to re-train the brain, and so we worked on trying to "pattern" Larry. This meant re-teaching him how to crawl using a different set of movements. In order to get Larry to do this, everyone in the family would get down on the floor and crawl to try to show him by example. The love and cooperation that this required really brought our family together. It was an amazing thing. We drove to Philadelphia every other week for about a year, but Larry didn't improve. Although we prayed for a miracle, none ever came. However, I would later come to believe that Larry himself actually was the miracle. He was a love child delivered to our family for a reason, and his presence caused something very special to happen between us — much love, respect and compassion.

"Destiny is not a matter of chance, it is a matter of choice."
— William Jennings Bryan

Life Lesson #6 - When Opportunity Knocks, Answer the Door:

This is one lesson I simply cannot stress enough. Most of the time in my life, I did answer the door when opportunity knocked, and the few regrets I have are when I didn't. Listen, of course you can't do everything, be everything and be everywhere (although I certainly tried). You need to make choices in life. But choices are for the victor. I always tried to make my choices based around the betterment of my family. If you can visualize it, you can make it better; or you have to find a way to make it work. Only you can fix your problems or accept them.

CHAPTER SEVEN
The Move Out West

"What you leave behind is not what is engraved in stone monuments, but what is woven into the lives of others."
— Pericles, Ancient Greek Statesman

1964 began as a year of sadness for us. We had to accept that our son was officially "retarded" and not getting better. President Kennedy had been shot the previous November, and my friend, Arthur Winarick of the Concord Hotel was dying. It seemed the only bright spot was that business was getting better and better, and I continued to look good in the eyes of the Perl Organization. Fritzie and I were invited to attend a convention in Florida sponsored by one of the many companies owned by the Perl Organization. While we were there, Mel Harris invited us to take a trip with him, Lou and Herman, in their private plane. We flew to Freeport, Grand Bahama Island, which back then consisted of a dirt landing strip and one hotel called The Caravel, which had 34 rooms. There was another hotel in the process of being built and the Perl Organization was a major investor. It was going to be called The Lucayan Beach Hotel. It was being constructed in Florida, floated over on barges and assembled on the island. What a sight. The imagination and vision that Lou, Herman, Mel and the team of architects and builders had was incredible. They constructed a city of everything you could dream of out of a sleepy fishing village. I knew then that in order to get any place in this world, you must be able to visualize an end goal and then do it. Imagination and dreams are necessary for success. Thanks again Mel. The trip and the lesson were invaluable.

> **Mini-Lesson:** *Imagination and dreams are necessary for success. Visualization is the stuff that dreams are made of. I learned to lead, follow or get out of the way.*

We went back home to Monticello where life was good for a while. But both Fritzie and I knew that it was time to make some changes, even though we didn't know which direction to take. Larry's condition still haunted us and we wanted to make sure that we were doing everything we could to help him. We spoke to a lot of people and found out about another program in Colorado Springs, Colorado, put together by a Dr. Lisa Gellner from London, England. She apparently had a retarded son of her own, and through her method of coaching and training had taught him to be self-sufficient enough to travel by himself and hold down a job, which back then, was not considered the norm. We also did not know how serious her son's condition was in comparison to Larry's, so it was very difficult to make an accurate comparison.

Sometime in 1965, I took a trip out to Colorado to see Dr. Gellner, armed with little more than a dream to see my little boy healthy and happy. I pleaded with her to accept Larry into her program, if for no other reason, than she did not have a child from New York State (or a Jewish child) in the program and we would do everything to help raise money and help the program grow. She agreed to have Larry join the program in 1966. I was so excited to fly home and share the news with my family. How utterly stupid I was in hindsight. The only thing we saw in our minds was the promise of a "normal" son. The sad truth is that if I had to do it all over again, I would. Just to make sure that I gave my son every chance possible to have a normal life, whatever I considered that to be. If it were you, what would you want your parents to do?

When I returned, we started to dismantle our lives. I told Herman Perl, Mel Harris and the folks at the Concord Hotel of our plans. We put our house up for sale, bought a new Chevy Caprice station wagon and broke the news to my parents, who were not too happy to find out that we were taking their beloved grandchildren across the country again. Fritzie's parents were not so unhappy, as we were moving closer to their neck of the woods. My staff and customers had a big party for me and presented me with a plaque wishing us good luck. I had arranged for my job to be filled by Danny Feldman, a cousin of Bob Soll, one of my dearest friends forever. Danny was an excellent stylist and a very good manager. Herman was very happy that I found Danny to run Beauty Industries, and I was very happy about doing the right thing before we left. Imagine, Danny's son Larry came back into my life many years later. He is a great guy and a successful businessman who is still in my life. It's all about doing the right thing. You never know how it's going to come back to you, but it always does.

> **Mini-Lesson:** *Always think about your name and reputation. Doing the right thing is everything.*

"If you tried to do something but couldn't, you are far better off than if you had tried to do nothing and succeeded."
— John T. Ragland, Jr.

Steve Lawrence and Eydie Gorme came to our "going away party" and gave us sterling silver coasters and a platter I still have to this day. They were all such warm and wonderful people. It was not easy to leave, but at the time we felt we had no choice. I arranged the rental of the U-Haul truck and trailer to drive to Colorado Springs on January 14, my birthday, which I considered a good omen. We sold our house within fourteen days, packed up our lives, loaded up our car, truck and trailer and left for the big move. Since we couldn't take the truck on some roads, we worked out a plan whereby Fritzie, Larry, Leslie, Lori, and Viola would take the shorter, Southern route with the car and I would take Steve and our dog, Snuggles on the roads across the middle of the country, where the truck had clearance, but we arranged our travel schedule so that we would all arrive in Colorado at about the same time.

We kissed and hugged goodbye at about 6pm, and we decided to drive through the night. Fritzie and I worked out a way to contact each other every night at the set time of 8:00 pm by calling my mother's house. Remember there were no cell phones back then. The plan was that Fritzie would call Mom "person to person" first and give my mother the number of the motel where she was staying. Then I would call mom "person to person" shortly after, get the number and call Fritzie to exchange our travel progress. Also in tow was a couple named Luther (Pierre) and Michel Popek, who had worked for me at the Concord and were visiting from Europe. They decided to join us for the cross-country drive and help me open up a beauty salon in Kaufman's Department

Store in Colorado Springs. I had arranged to build a salon in the department store through my networking. The Popeks were good friends, and we'd even hosted their wedding at our home. Luther planned to follow me in the 1964 Mercedes that he brought over from Germany. They were great stylists with a hot car.

In hindsight, it was an insane plan. It was a very cold night and after a few hours of driving, the snow was coming down pretty hard, although the roads were being cleared as we drove, so it wasn't as bad as you might imagine. Pierre and Michel had fallen behind somewhere, but we had a meeting place arranged up ahead. Then it happened — the truck broke down right on the highway. All the lights on the truck were out and the hazards weren't working either, so it seemed to be either a dead battery or the alternator. It was pitch black and I didn't have the foggiest idea where we were. We waited for someone to come by and help us for over an hour. No such luck. I decided to walk ahead with one of our two flashlights to hopefully find someone to give us a tow. I thought it was too dangerous to have Steve walk with me on the dark snowy road, so I gave him the other flashlight and told him to stay under the blankets with the dog and not to open the door for anyone but the police. Another insane plan.

After about two miles of running, I came to the next exit and saw a police car. At first the cop inside thought I was insane, because I was so happy to see him. I explained that I had left my son and dog two miles back in my dead U-Haul truck. He said I was nuts to be driving in the snow in the middle of the night, and that no cars had been on the road in hours. He told me to jump in, and we drove about ten minutes back toward the truck, while the policeman called for a tow truck to meet us there. When we arrived, Steve and the dog were gone. I went into total shock. The cop kept me standing up as my knees gave way and I began to sob. I became hysterical, running down the highway yelling for Steve. The policeman called in an all-points bulletin to be on the lookout for a boy and a dog. He tried to calm me down by saying that it didn't look like there was any foul play, and he was sure that we would find them. There was nothing I could do but sit in the police car, wait, pray and listen to the radio calls stating no boy was found. The tow truck finally came — it was probably only thirty minutes, but it truly seemed like days. I rode in the police car to the gas station two or three miles ahead. I couldn't believe that I had lost my son in Pennsylvania. I think the stress took ten years off my life. The next voice on the police radio sounded like the voice of God, "We have a boy and a dog ahead 10 miles." They were at the meeting place which Pierre, Michel and I had agreed to. It seemed that Pierre had stopped for gas and caught up with the truck which he saw on the side of the road. He said Steve and the dog were freezing, so he wrapped them up in his warm car and took them to the meeting place. I later asked him why he didn't leave me a note, and he replied, "I thought you would know it was us." I was so very happy and relieved that I quickly forgave him. But the trip had just begun.

> **Mini-Lesson:** *If you never make a mistake, you never make anything.*

I called U-Haul and they said no problem, they would give me a new truck — all I had to do was unload the one I was using and load the new one. "No Way," I said. It had taken four men and two boys ten hours to load everything we owned into the truck and trailer. They said if we stayed overnight, they would put their best mechanic to work on it all night. We stayed at a local motel, and they went to work on the truck. Around noon the next day, they told us they couldn't fix it. So we wound up having to unload and then reload it all anyway. It was 5pm by the time we hooked up the trailer and finally started out again. It was pretty crazy.

We drove about four hours and were nearing Toledo, Ohio, on the Ohio Turnpike when we stopped at a typical Howard Johnson-type rest stop. It was a large complex with the store on the left side of the building, bathrooms straight ahead, the restaurant to the right with a row of public phones in between. We all walked in together, sat down in the restaurant and ordered our dinner. I excused myself and walked to the washroom to splash some water on my face. I looked in the mirror at my own grubby, unwashed and unshaven face and chuckled to myself that I looked just like a typical truck driver at a truck stop on a run across the country, and I guess, at that point, I actually was. I was wearing jeans and a sweatshirt with my old Army fatigue jacket.

When I left the restroom I went right over to the phones, as I knew I was late for my check-in call to Mom and Fritzie. We made contact and I filled them in on the previous day's events. After assuring them that all was fine, we said our good-byes. Then just as I was hanging up the phone, this guy came out of nowhere from my right side, punched me square in the face and put a gun to my head! He was about 6'3" tall, 230 pounds and he looked like hell. I could immediately tell that there was something terribly wrong with this man. One thing I'll never forget were his eyes. When I looked into them I saw that they were fiery red and wild.

My reaction was so spontaneous it was as if I had practiced for the moment all my life. My head rolled with the punch but as I spun around, I knocked the gun out of his hand and broke his wrist at the same time. He screamed in pain, but tried to hit me again. My self-defense instincts kicked in and I must have punched him at least ten times right in the face. I think I broke the guy's jaw, nose and cheekbone, but despite that, he was in such a highly agitated state that he continued to come at me. So I used his momentum to throw him into a water cooler. It smashed on his head, and the water went all over the floor.

A crowd started to gather and I called for Pierre to help me. When he ran over and took in the scene, I remember him saying, "it looks like you're doing fine." Then the man started to get up again. This time I hit him with such force that he fell backwards, hit the floor and finally lay still, not moving. At the same moment a policeman ran into the restaurant, just in time to see me hitting this maniac and finally knocking him out. The cop threw me up against the phones, handcuffed me and took me to the police car. When I tried to explain what happened, he told me to shut up — that I would have plenty of time to tell my story. Two more police cars arrived and they all ran inside the restaurant.

When we got to the police station I tried to explain to the desk sergeant that I was moving from upstate New York on my way to Colorado with my family of six (who were nowhere to be seen). That my son was back at the Howard Johnson on the highway with another couple that we were traveling with, and that I was a good citizen, a businessman and a former military cop. The policeman didn't believe a word I was saying and was obviously losing his patience with me. Not so hard to believe when you consider what I must've looked like at the time — a dirty, bloody, unshaven guy in fatigues, who had just knocked a man out, and might have killed him. Then miraculously, it seemed, the other cops came rushing in with what looked like a busload of people, including Pierre and Michel and my son, Steve. They began to explain to both the sergeant and me the truly bizarre chain of events that led us all to this point.

The man who attacked me had escaped from a mental institution in Pennsylvania and hijacked a bus headed towards Chicago. He robbed all the people on the bus, putting their cash and jewelry in a big bag. The bus driver tried to contain the situation and told the crazy man that he needed to phone the main office of the bus company because if he didn't check in every four hours they'd send out the highway patrol to find the bus. Whether this was true or not, the guy believed it, and he told the driver to pull into the Howard Johnson's rest stop to make the call. The driver got off the bus and instead of calling his bus company, smartly made a frantic call to the police and then promptly hid. When he didn't return to the bus, the mental patient went searching the restaurant for him. That's when he saw me on the phone. I'm not sure if he thought I was the driver or if he just thought he'd rob one more person, but I was definitely a guy in the wrong place at the wrong time.

Mini-Lesson: *Never allow yourself to be bullied.*

When the police finally pieced all of this information together, they apologized for the mix up and commended me for being so courageous. They then drove me to the hospital, because I had broken my finger during the altercation and needed to get the cut on my face attended to. Unfortunately, the orthopedic guys were off duty that night so my finger wasn't set right, but I just wanted to get the hell out of there, so I decided I'd manage. For the rest of the trip, Steve had to help me drive by shifting the floor gear on the truck, essentially learning to drive a stick shift at age eight. (By the way, the finger never healed properly and it still looks broken to this day). The rest of the trip involved more bad weather but not nearly as much drama. We drove through Illinois and Indiana without incident, and basically skidded our way through Nebraska and Colorado all the while keeping in daily phone contact with Fritzie and the girls, although I left out the bad parts until we saw them in person, as I didn't want to worry them more than I already had. Thank God Fritzie and the girls' Southern route was smooth and uneventful.

> **Mini-Lesson:** *When you make a mistake admit it. The trip was a mistake.*

When we finally arrived in Colorado Springs, we set up temporary base camp at a local motel and went looking for a place to live. We found a great house that we loved on Clarkson Drive, with a front view of Pikes Peak and the Cheyenne Mountain Range, and a back view of Austin Bluffs — beautiful! The simple ranch house cost $24,000 and had a finished basement, five bedrooms and three baths. Thanks to another GI Mortgage and Fritzie's now highly developed homemaking skills, we thought we'd arrived at our little corner of paradise, all patched up and ready for our new life. We were a family again, with a house and a dream. We moved quickly to get the boys enrolled in school, making sure that Larry got settled into the special program at Dr. Gellner's Center.

I was able to conclude the deal with Kaufman's Department Store to open a beauty salon in their store. We did some renovations and the salon turned out to be a beautifully furnished and a very stylish spot. But unfortunately for us, sophistication hadn't reached the Rockies yet. The local women didn't get their hair cut or styled much. Long, natural hair was the style out west, and many of the women wore cowboy hats and ponytails. Even though the Air Force Academy and several other military facilities were the dominant local industries, at the time, Colorado

Springs still had a very small town atmosphere, and the salon was perhaps a bit ahead of its time for the area, except for the Broadmoor Hotel, a beautiful place with a very good beauty salon as our competition. Although those who did come to the salon became loyal customers, and we had enough money to pay our bills and make rent, the tips were pretty low, and I started to lose interest in the business quickly.

But I knew the most important reason we were in Colorado was to get Larry the best help we could. So Fritzie and I decided to get involved in the parents' groups at Larry's school, as we promised. We were welcomed with open arms, and I eventually became vice-president of the parents' association. It was a wonderful community and our neighbors were such nice people, inviting us to a seemingly endless rotation of dinners and parties. In an effort to build the business, I convinced two more hairstylists from the Concord to come out and work with us at Kaufman's Salon. So now in addition to Pierre and Michel staying with us, we also put Don and Karen up at our place. I tried everything to increase business — newspaper ads, radio, lectures, even doing hair at the Miss Colorado beauty contest, but nothing seemed to make much of a difference. Business was slow, and slow was not a good thing.

Then my Mom and Dad came out to visit with the intention of possibly moving out permanently, as they missed us and especially their grandbabies. It was incredible to watch the tremendous love my parents had for their grandchildren. I prayed that I would be even half as good a grandparent as they were with our kids. I told my dad that we would find him a nice building to manage or be a superintendent. He would have a nice place to live, some money in his pocket and the chance to utilize his talent to fix, repair and build things.

He was 62 and still not adjusting well to his forced retirement from the Star Corrugated factory in Maspeth Queens, NY, so I thought this would be a good move for him. But sadly, just eleven days after he arrived in Colorado, my dad suffered a heart attack while playing with Larry in the kids' room. Fritzie ran to give him mouth-to-mouth resuscitation while I called for an ambulance. On the way to the hospital, right before he left this world, Dad told me to take care of my mother. I knew what that meant, and Mom would wind up living with us for the majority of the next 27 years. Isn't that what you're supposed to do?

Mom and I flew home to Brooklyn with Dad's body on a commercial flight for a proper burial and to sit shiva with the family in NY, while Fritzie stayed in Colorado with the kids. After making arrangements for the burial, I hoped that at least some people would come to the funeral to show respect, but I got the most wonderful shock of my life — there must have been 400 people that came to the funeral home and almost 150 cars at the cemetery in Queens. Dad might not have been the most successful in business, he may have only earned just enough for his limited needs and he didn't have a lot of possessions, but he sure did something right in his life.

The people who spoke at the service (most of whom I had never met) said the most wonderful words a son would ever want to hear about his father. Harry truly cared about and helped many of the people he came in contact with, and they all appreciated and respected him immensely. Although I always loved and respected my Dad, I believe that you never really understand the value of someone you love until you no longer have them in your life. Sad, but often true. He was always such a kind man and a hard worker, not only to his family, but to just about everyone he encountered. At that moment, I was even more proud to be his son. I treasure my memories of him, which have always kept me in a positive mode.

> **Mini-Lesson:** *Life isn't always fair but it's still good. When you cry, cry with someone — it's more healing than crying alone. Never underestimate the value that a parent can give. My Dad knew how much I loved him and I thank him for letting me dream.*

My family was very sad, but we all had no choice but to adjust to life without Poppa Harry. My mom decided to leave Brooklyn and come to live with us in Colorado, and the world's most patient and kind daughter-in-law, Fritzie, made all the necessary arrangements. Mom officially became the newest addition to our family, and the children loved having their grandmother around. Life went on. The business, though not spectacular, was still alive and I continued to do what I could to further it along.

One day I received a call from Jane Morgan, one of my very special clients from New York. She was a world-class singer who made a string of big hits including the song, "Fascination" as well as the popular, "Hey Big Spender." Jane asked if I would be interested in designing a salon for a friend of hers. The friend was Bill Harrah of the famous Harrah's Hotel & Casino. I gladly agreed. Jane also asked if I would be willing to do her hair for an upcoming opening of Harrah's in Reno, Nevada. I told her that wherever she needed me, I'd be there. Jane was a lovely person and a wonderful friend, but I also knew that with her many connections, she was certainly an important person to be connected with. Her husband, Jerry Weintraub, was a great agent and promoter as well as a really good guy to me. I'm so grateful that they have been in my life.

Mr. Harrah made arrangements for me to come up to Reno where he was building a hotel atop his casino. He also wanted me to check out his smaller, more exclusive hotel for high rollers in beautiful Lake Tahoe. Mr. Harrah was an interesting guy. He was a huge sports enthusiast, with a penchant for fine cars. His massive antique car collection was easily one of the largest and finest in the world. I had a good time and worked hard for Mr. Harrah, laying out salons at both hotels and getting a nice paycheck for it. By the way, one of my most memorable moments was having Bill Harrah drive me from Reno up to Lake Tahoe in his Lamborghini. It was my first time in a car like that. My body was basically lying flat with just my head propped up. Bill was going so fast along the narrow, winding roads that we made the trip in under an hour. I didn't think we were going to make it. At the time, there were no guard rails and I thought we were going to go over the mountain the whole time. Just a bit scary, to say the least.

I spent a day or two getting the salons looking great on paper and found a lift back to Reno from a hotel employee in a slow, safe shuttle van. Bill Harrah was a great guy and treated me very well during my time in Reno and Tahoe. He was known for his warmth and good relations with both his customers and employees and was the first to invite African-American entertainers to perform at his casinos. In fact, the main theater in Harrah's Reno was named Sammy's Showroom after the fabulous Sammy Davis, Jr. Bill broke tradition by hiring employees regardless of skin color or gender, and his was one of the first casinos to employ women as dealers.

California Here We Come

"The journey of a thousand miles starts with a single step."
— Chinese Proverb

It was time to return to Colorado Springs, but I was not very excited about that. Dr. Lisa Gellner, the woman who ran Larry's school and research center, had passed away, making it a very sad and confusing time for us. The program she created began to drift into limbo. We did not really see any improvement with Larry or any of the other children in the program either. It had been a dream of ours to see our son normal, but it did not seem like this was to be. We realized that we would have to leave the beautiful Colorado Rockies and look for another place to create his future, as well as ours, before we went completely broke, and it was getting very close. Around the same time, our wonderful nanny, Viola, found and married a great guy she met in a church group, and they moved to California to make their new life together. We were sad to see Viola go, but we could not have been happier for her.

Mini-Lesson: *Never stop trying and never give up.*

We decided to also go to California to see if we could make any sort of life for ourselves in Los Angeles or on the West Coast in general. Fritzie and I had some family there, and as always, a positive attitude and sense of adventure took us on our way to the next chapter of our lives. We put our house up for sale and closed the salon. Pierre, Michel, Don, and Karen all went to work at the beautiful Broadmoor Hotel in Colorado Springs and we wished them well. We packed up everything we needed into a small trailer, hooked it up to the car and started off towards the first leg of our next journey, Alamosa, Colorado, to visit some of Fritzie's family. Fritzie had four sisters and a brother who were scattered in Colorado, Texas, Utah, Oregon and California. When we got to Alamosa, we traded our dog, Snuggles, for Fritzie's niece Katy, who was around 12 years old at the time. We all thought it was a great idea to have Katy travel with us to see the country and also be able to help us out with watching the children when needed.

Fritzie and I agreed that we would need to conserve funds on this trip. She had done a lot of camping growing up and convinced me that camping out during our trip was a good way to economize. So, before we left Colorado we bought a slew of camping equipment including lanterns, a small battery-powered refrigerator, Coleman stove, flashlights, etc., and made arrangements to stay in different, campsites, cabins, cottages and state parks along the way. We arrived at Mesa Verde, Colorado at dusk, but when we tried to settle into the cabin we had rented, it was already occupied — by a grizzly bear! We screamed and ran back to the car, not sure if we should laugh or cry. It was pitch black out and I was not brave enough to venture back in to see if we scared the bear away, so we drove to the Administrator's office but they were closed for the evening and there was no one there.

We wound up staying in a nearby motel for the night. So much for our first foray into nature.

Mom was shaken up the most. The only bears she had ever seen in Brooklyn were at the Prospect Park Zoo, behind nice strong steel fences. The next morning we got up early to take in the beauty of the area and ask for our money back for the room we rented with the bear in it. We never did not get the money back, but we toured the Native American cliff dwellings, amazed at how they built their homes right into the mountain. "Probably so the bears wouldn't bother them," we all laughed. When it was time to leave Mesa Verde, we were all satisfied that we had seen a part of history and learned a few things — including a lesson to ask to see the cabin rooms before paying.

> **Mini-Lesson:** *Where you are is important, but not as important as where you are going.*

Our next stop was the breathtaking Grand Canyon. We arrived at the Grand Canyon State Park at dusk and drove to our assigned spot to make camp. Convincing my Mom that the bear episode was a fluke was not easy, but I guess she thought that this location was worth the risk of another possible encounter with wildlife. Our next problem was that I couldn't get a fire started on the Coleman stove. Not being an outdoorsman, what did I know from a Coleman stove? Fritzie and the kids were off to the restrooms, so I went to the tent next door and made a "knock, knock" noise with my mouth. I excused myself for intruding and asked the man at the "door" for help. He was quite nice and got the fire going for us right away. We settled in trying to cook our dinner. I bought steaks instead of hamburgers (which would have been much easier), which we overcooked and were not great. Oy, another lesson learned.

As darkness descended, it suddenly seemed that every single bug in Grand Canyon State Park had been waiting to suck me and my mom's blood. For some reason, the bugs didn't go after Fritzie and the kids, but Mom and I looked like we were doing a dance of slaps. Although the kids were disappointed, we couldn't get away from this world-famous natural wonder fast enough. We packed everyone up, shoved everything back in the trailer and put all of the camping equipment away, never to be used again. Needless to say, we wound up staying only at motels and hotels for the rest of the trip (preferably 2nd floor accommodations). Guess you can take the mother and son out of Brooklyn, but....

The next day, we all got a good look at that great big hole in the ground — the Grand Canyon. It was so beautiful and majestic that it took our breath away. We stopped for one night in Vegas, where we saw Jane Morgan's name on the marquee. We went to see her show and took Mom. It was very exciting and she treated us with great love. Mom thought it was a dream. Thanks Jane and Jerry. Then we started for California in search of our new home and, we hoped, our new life. The kids were behaving great- singing songs and playing the "count the different cars" game, but about halfway to Los Angeles, in the middle of the desert, our air conditioner broke. As you could imagine, crossing the hot desert with eight complaining people in a cramped, hot station wagon was not a helluva lot of fun, but we finally made it. We dropped my mom off at her sister Bea's apartment in Beverly Hills and then we visited Fritzie's sister, Darlene, who let us stay at her house.

We spent five days there, having a great time, getting sunburned and looking for that special job, or sign — or something. I found out that I couldn't work as a hairstylist because of the very strict California state licensing requirements that would've taken me almost a year to complete. I was looking at everything with an eye toward making a living but nothing clicked. Although I had made many appointments in California through my many friendships and connections, I had no real job opportunities and nothing felt right. We left for San Francisco where we stayed at a motel with bugs. One bright spot was running into Buddy Maurice's family, vacationing from Miami Beach, while sightseeing. We all had lunch together, caught up on old times, including wonderful memories of the Fontainebleau Hotel and my start in hairstyling. Then we parted ways.

We decided to check out of our hotel and head up to Lake Tahoe to enjoy the beauty of the drive and the cooler weather of the high altitude. Everything was so clean and green, and we fell in love with the Sierras and the crystal clear Lake Tahoe, where I had visited alone the year before. I was so happy to share it with my family this time. We stayed for two days and got ready for the last major stop of the trip, Salt Lake City. We had an easy drive over to Utah, and were excited to visit the famous temple and hear the Mormon Tabernacle Choir. The thought was so exhilarating that we just had to sing during our drive. We didn't know any Mormon songs, so the music from the Sound of Music had to do. We were disappointed upon arrival at the temple to hear that non-Mormons were not able to visit or hear the choir. Even though Fritzie's mom and Katy's family were all Mormon, we still didn't qualify. We did some sightseeing, and enjoyed the scenic mountain range surrounding the city. Then we dropped off Katy in Alamosa, picked up Snuggles the dog and headed home to Colorado sad and still looking for the magic.

Upon our return, we decided it was now time to head back to our safe haven, New York and we began the now familiar preparations. We sold our house quickly and cheaply, called a moving company, packed up all of our belongings, and said our goodbyes, but before we left, we sat down and to make some important family decisions. Mom said that she wanted to go to California for a while to live with a friend who lived in the same building as her sister, Bea. Although we knew we'd miss her, we thought it was a good move for her at the time. So we saw Mom off on a plane to Los Angeles, where we had arranged for Cousin Ira and Barbara to receive her, wishing her love and luck and promising that we'd continue to help support her.

Fritzie flew back to New York to conduct an advance search for a place to live and it was decided that she would stay with my brother and his family for a few days in Rockville Center on Long Island. The kids and I had a nice (and this time, thankfully uneventful) drive back to New York, but when we met up with Fritzie, she was very upset. When I asked what was wrong, she told me she was very uncomfortable staying at my brother's house because he had said to her, "Please don't let Larry wander around outside. We don't want anyone to know we've got a retarded child like Larry in our family."

Wow. I know I must've turned white with anger and rage. It would have hurt less if he had hit me right in the face with a hammer. On that day, I picked up Fritzie from my brother's house and never looked back. I found (and still find) it hard to believe that anyone could say something so ignorant and hurtful, especially to a family member. But it happens. And although I'm pretty sure that he and his family regretted saying it over the years, I never wanted to be involved with my brother again. And I never forgot. Ironically, my brother passed away a couple of years ago, and I took Larry with me to his funeral. I didn't want anyone to think that I did the wrong thing by not attending, so I went to see him off — with his beautiful nephew, Larry, beside me.

> **Mini-Lesson:** *Everything can change in the blink of an eye. But don't worry, God never blinks. Don't compare your life to others; you have no idea what their journey is all about.*

Fritzie, the kids and I found a motel on Sunrise Highway in Long Island to spend the night, but after checking our resources, we realized that we couldn't stay for very long. Money was a major problem. Colorado had eaten up most of our funds, and we were just about broke. We had only $300 left to our name, and in ten days the moving truck was set to arrive with our belongings, but we had no place to unload our stuff. Just another day in the life of the Levines.

Life Lesson #7 - Nothing is More Constant Than Change:

There's no crime in trying, but there are regrets in not trying. We went to Colorado and then California in an effort to make things better for our family, and we sacrificed a lot in our quest for something more. It turned out it wasn't our end destination, and it didn't necessarily turn out as we had expected. However, we tried. Whether it's in business, health matters or anything else, if it doesn't feel right, change it. And even if (or when) you lose, don't lose the lesson. People who are satisfied with their current position in life will probably stay there. But those who really believe they can do better will always move ahead. Life moves on and so should you.

Part Two

CHAPTER EIGHT
Back Home in New York

LIFE LESSON #8...

LIFE REALLY IS BEAUTIFUL: PEOPLE CAN BE GREAT WHEN GIVEN THE OPPORTUNITY

"Good works are links that form a chain of love."
— Mother Teresa.

I called an old friend I'd worked with at the salon in Great Neck named Enrico to see if he could help. Enrico and his wife, JoAnna, had five small children and lived in a big old house in Great Neck, Long Island. When I shared our predicament with him, he generously offered his home to us. I hadn't seen nor talked to Enrico for five years and he was financially strapped himself. But he made room for us in his home and showed extreme kindness to my family and me. It was a perfect example of the goodness of someone's heart. Thank you, my friend, for taking my family in and for making us feel like family. Grateful isn't a good enough word for what you did. What you may or may not have realized is that you saved our lives.

We looked and looked for a house and finally found a great one in Wantagh, a nice town on the south shore of Long Island. It wasn't too expensive and was close to everything we needed. The only problem was the house was $33,000 and we didn't have the required G.I. bill down payment of $3,000. I called my childhood friend, Bob Soll, who also lived in Wantagh, and he convinced his dad to loan us the money. I promised to pay it back as soon as I could, and that was good enough for them. I did pay it back, and Harry didn't even charge me any interest. I'll always be thankful to Harry and Bob Soll for taking a chance on me — you were both such wonderful and generous souls. It just goes to show you that if you don't ask, how are you going to find out the possibilities available? Life really is beautiful and people are great when given the opportunity to help. Sometimes you just have to ask.

Unbelievably, when the moving truck arrived, we were ready to unload. Thank God I paid that bill before we left Colorado. We moved out of Enrico's house and moved once again into a new home and fresh surroundings. We began to settle in, and once again Fritzie fixed up the new house, making it a home. That meant that I had to start bringing home the bacon — quickly. My family needed to eat. There was $300 between starvation and us. The only thing we had going for us is that we believed. There is always a choice between fear and trepidation vs. the "I think I can" approach. For us, the latter prevailed. Fritzie and I were determined to make ends meet and didn't even consider the alternative. So we did what we had to do. We worked harder.

> **Mini-Lesson:** *"Twenty years from now you will be more disappointed by the things you didn't do than by the ones you did do. So throw off the bowlines. Sail away from the safe harbor. Catch the trade winds in your sails. Explore. Dream. Discover."* — **Mark Twain**

Before we left Colorado, I was introduced to a pair of brothers (the Springfield Brothers) who had invented a car wash machine called the "Robo-Wash." I was intrigued by the concept and saw it as a great residual income business. After a few meetings with them, I mentioned that I was planning to move back East and wondered if they'd be interested in allowing me to franchise their technology. They agreed, and from then on, I guess I was in the car wash business — contingent on finding some franchisees, of course. Armed with a business card that now had a Long Island address, I went out looking for business. But since it was not a business that provided real income instantly, I decided to do hair once again to pay the bills. I got a job at a salon in Manhasset on the north shore of Long Island called Megaris of Athens. It was owned by two very nice Greek brothers who let me work Thursday through Saturday, the busiest days in the salon business.

But Long Island is an expensive place to live, so I called an old friend, Stuart Stern, who I heard was selling life insurance for a living. Stuart told me that he thought I could make a lot of money doing the same and he kindly introduced me to his boss. He offered me a job selling insurance Monday through Wednesday mornings. The boss would take me to some bad neighborhoods in Brooklyn where he told me to knock on doors in apartment buildings and try to sell insurance. I didn't really enjoy it, particularly because of the neighborhoods I was covering. But knowing what I know now, I think that if I'd really applied myself, I probably would have gotten pretty darn good at it by approaching selling from a much different perspective.

In any event, I accepted the arrangement but continued working in the beauty salon the rest of the week. Plus I was still trying to sell the car washes whenever I could. Through another connection, I was also able to get yet another job at a nightclub in New York City as a front doorman and bouncer on Friday and Saturday nights where I collected money at the door and helped out with any problems. So I was now holding down four jobs at one time. I'm not sure how I did it (or how my eyes stayed open while driving from one job to another) but I did. And I do believe that anyone who wants to, can.

One important thing that got me through it was knowing that it wouldn't last forever. I finally started to make a couple of Robo-Wash sales, and before long I had enough to think about opening my own salon. I found the perfect location in Great Neck then called Enrico and offered him a 25% partnership in M. Walter Hairstylist and he agreed. With the help of another great friend, Mr. B (Burt Lipman - better known throughout the country as Mr. B's Beauty Equipment and Supplies), whom I had known from the Concord, we were able to get the necessary materials and we were open for business.

We still had a great reputation in the area (from five years prior) and it didn't take long for business to pick up. However, it seemed that my family's financial needs were becoming greater too. Whatever I brought in just never seemed to be enough. One of the reasons we chose to live on Long Island was that they had one of the best programs available for Larry. We got him into in a great facility called the Center for the Emotionally Disturbed in Syosset, New York. Larry was picked up daily at 8:30am and returned home at 4pm. He seemed to be doing well and we had him evaluated as often as possible to make sure we explored anything and everything that could possibly be of benefit to him. With the expenses of the new business as well as the cost of Larry's program, I had no choice but to let the macho image I had of myself go and accept that I needed help. So Fritzie and I discussed the possibility of her going back to work, which was something that hadn't been necessary for over a decade. She got a job as a part-time X-ray technician at Long Beach Hospital, while also working two days a week in a private doctor's office in order to help us make it through our latest financial challenge. You do what you have to do.

In order for Fritzie to work, we needed to get someone to help with the children, so we hired a housekeeper named Brenda through the same agency in New York City we got Viola from. I didn't pay attention to her last name until about a week after we hired her. Steve, who was nine at the time, stayed home sick from school that day. Fritzie and I went off to work and left Steve in the care of our new housekeeper. He kept getting up to go to the bathroom and was constantly sent back to bed by Brenda. He told her that he wanted to stay in our bedroom so he could be close to the bathroom and watch television on our bed. She sternly sent him back to his room, saying, "You shouldn't spread sickness." Steve obeyed and went back to his room, while she proceeded to clean our house. And I don't mean clean the dirt. I mean she cleaned us out. That's right, she packed all of Fritzie's clothes right down to the underwear, stockings, shoes, coats, jewelry — everything. She left my clothes, but took my jewelry as well.

We didn't have a lot, but Brenda took it all, including a medal that Fritzie's Dad was awarded in World War I. She packed everything in boxes and apparently took four trips to the post office to ship everything home to North Carolina, telling Steve she was going shopping for us. When my son called Fritzie and told her that Brenda left and never came back, Fritzie drove home, saw what had happened and called me up hysterical. I came home immediately and called the police. They checked with the cab company and the post office and were able to recover some of the boxes, which hadn't been shipped yet — the ones that contained clothes, mostly underwear. She got away with all of our luggage and whatever was packed into it.

The police told us that Brenda Outlaw was the only one in her family from North Carolina that didn't have a record. That's right, her name was Brenda Outlaw! I guess she now officially fit right in with the rest of them. Starting over was nothing new to us, but the one thing that hurt more than anything was that it was right around Christmas time, and Brenda Outlaw also took the few presents we had under the tree. It obviously didn't make for a great Christmas. But we survived. We got beyond it because we wanted to and because we had to. And as always, our family was our salvation.

Luckily, the next year passed fairly uneventfully. Our children made some wonderful friends in the new neighborhood; they loved school and were fully participating in the extracurricular activities of the community. They seemed to be enjoying their own lives very much. I had left my other jobs to concentrate on the beauty salon and the car washes since I thought that these had the most earning potential. The salon was doing well, although my heart wasn't really in it. I did still enjoy the satisfaction of helping clients, and as always, Enrico was a great partner.

But as fate would have it, the following Christmas Eve while having dinner with my family after a long, hard day and looking forward to the busiest week of the year in salon bookings, I got a phone call from the Great Neck Police telling me that the salon was on fire. I went crazy and drove back to Great Neck at 75 miles per hour to see what was going on. It seemed that a fire started in the restaurant next door and all the storefronts on our side of street burned down entirely, putting us all out of business. I cried, and I cried deeply. It was a long while since I'd felt that level of despair.

But on Christmas Day, I decided to contact Peter Coppola who had worked with me at Marvin's Hairstylist six years earlier. He owned and operated Peter's Place, the beauty salon right around the corner from ours, and our biggest competition. He went on to be very successful in the business, opening many salons and creating a very well known brand. Peter kindly made room for me and my staff to work in his salon until after the first of the year so we could honor all of our appointments. He didn't charge for the space although he did take 50% of our fees, which I thought was a fair deal for both of us. Peter was a real pro and had a wonderful way with people. And with that, we did what we had to do, and made it through the holidays — all the while, making sure to take care of the customer.

Life Lesson #8 - Life Really is Beautiful; People Can Be Great When Given the Opportunity:

All the security, benefits, and mental comfort that I worked so hard to achieve was gone. I felt disoriented and was more than a little concerned about our future. It was certainly a time to reevaluate where my life was and where I'd come from. I had come a long way and experienced enormous highs as well as extremely sad lows. But for the first time I started to doubt my abilities and judgment — and it wouldn't be the last. However, as shattered as it was, I never lost sight of my goals and long term plan, which was to win and build a future for my family and myself. I had to gather all my strength to pick myself up, dust myself off, and do the right thing. I believe the key is that I was able to visualize myself on the other side of success and I never allowed myself to lose sight of that. We are all in a common bond of struggle in this life. Compassion is the great key in making it bearable — if you use it.

Nothing in life is easy, but look around you. Even when things seem especially hopeless, there are glimmers of beauty and kindness all around you — I guarantee it. For every Brenda Outlaw, there is an Enrico, or one of the many other kind souls who opened their hearts to me and my family throughout the years. In fact, people never cease to amaze me. Those who go out of their way to help others have been my salvation as well as my inspiration.

CHAPTER NINE
Walter's ABCDs of Sales

LIFE LESSON #9...

IT'S NOT MAGIC, JUST WORK
HARDER THAN EVERYONE ELSE IF
YOU WANT TO SUCCEED

"Tomorrow is now."
— Eleanor Roosevelt

1969 - Wantagh, Long Island

*W*hen the holidays were over and I had finished with the insurance company, the adjusters and my bills, I realized that I was not in a position to rebuild unless I was willing to get into great debt. I knew that I didn't have the same feeling for the business anymore. I think that my experience in Colorado really took away my passion for hairstyling and makeup, and when you stop loving something, you don't do it as well as when you do. It became clear to me that it was probably time to move on. All of the exposure I had to successful businessmen over the years made me realize that there were other ways to be successful, and I was now ready to take my chances in the business world.

One of my salon clients tried to help me by introducing me to the Osrow family. The Osrows were two brothers, Leonard and Harold, whose company had invented the windshield ice scraper. Their company was expanding and they were interested in buying a Miami based company called Moonshine Car Wash. And after hearing about me from my client, they were also interested in me. So they requested a meeting and it went great. One meeting turned into several, and after some discussions, they offered me the chance to run Moonshine for them. I would get 25% of the company in stock, with the ability to convert that stock into Osrow Products stock, which was valued at $12 per share at the time. I would also get a salary, bonus and expenses paid. I don't know what they saw in me at that moment, but I was sure glad that they did. My confidence level hit the roof at a very difficult time in my life. I knew I could do it, just like the Little Engine That Could, and I truly believed that I would. So I let the Springfield Brothers know that I would no longer be pursuing Robo-Wash and they wished me good luck.

I hired a secretary and based myself out of a new office in Glen Cove, Long Island and then I went down to Miami to start the takeover of Moonshine Car Wash, a great name for a simple product. The concept was to sell soap and wax in 55-gallon drums on a monthly basis (residual income) to car dealerships that bought and installed the Moonshine Machine. The machine, which easily fit into a bay at the dealership, would thoroughly clean a car within a three-minute cycle. At my suggestion, the dealerships could now offer customers a clean car after their service, and of course, a clean car always runs better, right? The dealership owners and managers loved it and most importantly, so did the customers. It was a win-win situation all around.

I spent three to four days a week on the road selling the Moonshine service in different cities in the U.S., Canada, and Mexico. Fritzie and I weren't exactly prepared for all my time away and it was tough on the family, but I was always home for the weekends. Success was starting to happen — I could feel it. I would fly out every Monday to a different location and I started to get into a routine. When I arrived at the airport, I'd rent a car, go to a local motel, check-in, unpack and then look through the local phone book to see where the car dealerships were. I would go down the list in the yellow pages (we didn't have computers back then) and start making calls to get appointments with the owners. When I arrived at a dealer that I arranged a meeting with, I'd show them a video of the product and its benefits in action. Then I'd share letters from satisfied customers. In some cases, the owners knew the other owners and would call them to ask their opinion, so there was no room for any "B.S." on my part or anyone else's. While the mechanics were installing the mobile Moonshine machine, I would bring other managers in from other dealerships to see the car wash in action. Some thought it was a waste of time but others saw it as a time management and cost control benefit, as well as a value-added service for their customers. I would sell about 50% of the people I saw, which was a pretty darned good sales ratio.

I was able to sell 880 car washes to new car dealers in the first 2 ½ years and I'll always be grateful to the Osrow Family for funding my car wash career for those couple of years. All in all, I had a good relationship with the Osrow family and Harold and his wife, Laura. Harold passed away in the mid-1990s, and I remain friends with Laura today. I try to never let go of the quality people in my life, as they're very hard to come by. One of the main reasons I think that Harold Osrow liked me was that I didn't come up with excuses. I did my work with gusto and was grateful for the opportunity to be a partner and build a company.

But, things changed. Unable to leave a good thing alone, the engineers at the factory making the car wash devices began tinkering with the product in an effort to make it "better." What they wound up doing changed the concept of something elegantly simple to something very complicated, and as a result they made things better for our competitors, not us. Too many engineering bells and whistles caused more malfunctions, which led to more service calls on the new units. This obviously started to eat up money and time for both Moonshine and its customers, and it had a ripple effect on sales, as current customers weren't willing to recommend us anymore. Unfortunately, my 25% control couldn't override the decisions that led to these problems, and it didn't seem like things were going to change. So although we were wonderfully entrenched in Long Island with great friendships and relationships that are still in part of my life, I had no choice but to start thinking about my next move and a different future for myself.

> **Mini-Lesson: Learn to profit from your mistakes. If you can't, your competition will. Making a living should never be confused with making a life.**

Bahama Bound

> *"Some men see things and say 'why'?*
> *I dream of things that never were and ask, 'why not?'*
> *— John F. Kennedy*

It was around that time that I received a phone call from Harold Blair who was my friend from the Perl family, and the vice president of the Perl Organization. He asked how the family was doing, and wondered why he hadn't heard from me since I arrived back in New York. For some reason I didn't contact Herman Perl, Harold Blair or any of the friends that I had made while I ran the beauty salons. I guess the truth of the matter was that in my mind I believed that they knew me as a winner, and coming back from Colorado with no money and in a new business, wasn't exactly how I wanted them to see me. I wanted to head back towards the top before contacting them again.

But I was warmed to hear that Herman and Harold cared enough to keep abreast of my situation and progress through mutual friends. So when Harold invited me to lunch with him at the New Jersey office, I thought it was to catch up on old times and perhaps brag about what was happening at the Perl Corporation. When I arrived, much to my delight and surprise, he mentioned that Herman wanted me back in the business with him and asked if I would be interested in opening up and managing an office in Suffolk County, Long Island, to sell real estate in the Bahamas.

> **Mini-Lesson:** *Opportunity is knocking — open the door!*

Wow, I certainly didn't see that coming. I immediately told Harold that I was really excited about the offer and told him that if the money could be worked out, I was not only interested, but I thought that I'd love it! After I said that, he took me into Herman's office where I got the welcome of a returning son with a big hug and kiss and lots of promises of success. From that moment on, I never looked back. I came home and told Fritzie of my great meeting. We were both beyond excited. Another door opened because of relationships. Life can really be GREAT that way. Keep as many doors open as possible — you never know who is listening and watching.

Next, I met with Harold Osrow to tell him of my future plans. I assured him that I would stay as long as necessary to pass the torch and train my replacement. The board tried to convince me to stay on. I was flattered, and laughed when they teased me about selling land "underwater," but not before I corrected them, explaining that the land I'd be selling was most definitely "by the water" not under it. We all parted as friends six weeks later, and my new life was about to begin. Now all I had to do was to deliver, and with the complete belief that I was born to win, I knew that I could and would.

> **Mini-Lesson:** *Every day is a great day. Try listening to Frank Sinatra's "That's Life" and Sammy Davis Jr.'s "I Gotta Be Me" to get yourself in the right mindset.*

Harold Blair set up a meeting with me and Howard Beck, a big, robust man who was the sales manager for the New York City office. He was a born leader and a very talented salesman. He proceeded to explain to me how the business worked. Howard or his assistant would give a "front talk." This is when you stand up in front of a group of people without a podium to explain the virtues of owning land. In this case, specifically land in the Bahamas. It was just like any other prospecting business — you had to study and know the product inside out because the questions from the crowd ranged from the sublime to the ridiculous. No matter, you'd better have the right answer or else you'll lose credibility (and the sale) — fast.

After training with Howard for three months and helping to make several sales we became great friends, and we still are to this day. I was asked to visit Grand Bahama Island and see the place for myself. So Fritzie and I flew down. "My God!" I said when we landed. We both could not believe our eyes. The growth that had occurred since the last time we were there in 1964, when the Caravel Hotel with its 34 rooms was the only hotel on the island, was staggering. Now the hotels were many and there were several golf courses. They had actually cut the island in half to create more waterfront property — mind-boggling! I was beyond excited. What an opportunity!

The beauty of the landscaping and the architecture was incredible, and the people of the Bahamas were great – warm and open with wonderful attitudes. They are family. I knew that this was going to be an easy sale. Jeez, I was sold. I bought two pieces of property for myself right on the spot, which I was able to pay out over time. I learned quickly and was more than excited to dive right in, but there was one small catch: I had to have a full broker's license in order to sell real estate and be a manager, but I wasn't going to let that stop me. So as soon as we came home, I studied and trained for the real estate broker's license exam and within a month I took it and passed on the first try. Yeah!

> **Mini-Lesson:** *You can't be what you can't visualize.*
> *Try it!*

Birth of a Salesman

Harold Blair assigned me to the Nassau County, Long Island office for a short time where I worked with Danny Feldman (who I had hired to replace me at Beauty Industries). His son Larry is a great young man who runs 1500 successful Subway franchises in the United States. Talk about success. I am very proud of him, and glad we're friends today and staying involved in life together. Then we were off to the Bahamas Realty Convention at the Holiday Inn on the Grand Bahama Island, which was like the Academy Awards for the business, and a huge spectacle. The awards, the prizes, the bonuses, and the outfits — it was all larger than life. Sitting at Herman's table during dinner, I turned to him and said, "You know what I like about you?" "No, what?" he responded. "Everything!" I said. "And I promise you there will never be another convention that I won't be a winner at." Herman looked at me, nodded and said, "Somehow I knew you'd say that."

While I was there at the convention, I also had the opportunity to meet Jay Levan, from the Chicago office. He was a short, bald, heavyset man who looked more like Lou Costello's cousin than a real estate salesman. Jay was there celebrating his fifth year as the number one salesman in the entire company of over 2000 salesmen worldwide. I decided to find out what made him number one. I strode up to Jay, too focused on my question to be nervous. After I perfunctorily introduced myself, I pointedly asked, "So Mr. Levan, what makes you different? Do you have some sort of magic secret?" To which he calmly replied, "There's no magic, kid. I just work harder than anyone else. I'm not just a pretty face, you know." On that note, he smiled, turned around and walked away. I never forgot those words.

> **Mini-Lesson:** *The greatest tragedy in business is not that you tried and failed — but that you failed to try.*

When we returned five days later, Herman wired $10,000 into an account and told me to rent office space, get phones, hire a secretary, put ads in the paper for salesmen and arrange with restaurants for client sales meetings. He said he'd take care of the mailings, brochures and films. He also gave me a set of records that he produced on "Selling by Numbers." They are still a cherished memento of mine and I think that many, if not all, of the sales concepts covered in them still apply. I'd play the records through, one by one, listening intently. Then I'd listen to each one again with a note pad in hand and jot down questions I had as well as any tips that I thought were especially relevant. Finally, I'd listen a third time. Usually then, the answers to the questions that I had jotted down previously would all come to me.

> **Mini-Lesson:** *Learning how to learn according to your own style is one of the most important lessons in life. What's your learning style?*

One of the major points from the records that struck me at the time was that 80-90% of sales are made by 10% of the sales force. I realized that a true salesperson is a special breed of cat, a dynamic force that never lets fear enter his (or her) world, as they know that fear can stop them, and they DO NOT ALLOW ROADBLOCKS. They are enthusiastic, they genuinely enjoy seeing people and they tell the truth about what they sell. "The Professional," the salesman's salesman, is the mightiest Caesar of them all. That's what Herman called me, and I worked hard to prove him right. His sales program also talked about how getting your customer to buy is only half the battle. Getting them to buy YOU is the fundamental element to what he called "heart to heart selling."

Herman Perl was an amazing businessman, the best salesperson I ever met and a caring, wonderful human being. He made it all work together and left quite a legacy. Herman was also a great family man. He adored his wife, Ruth and their four children, and made a practice of intertwining his own family with his working family seamlessly. His brother, brother-in-law, cousins, and anybody that wanted to work hard and build something would have an opportunity to be part of it.

It was really from Herman that I started to piece together my own philosophy on sales and on life (which, of course, is reflected in this book's title). I began to realize, largely through Herman's incredible tutelage, that I was in the business of not just selling, but of helping people. In this particular case, I was helping people save money for their retirement using real estate as an investment for their future and/or a place to retire.

I rented space in a building at 330 Motor Parkway in Hauppauge, Long Island, hired Joyce, a terrific Gal Friday, got all the necessary office equipment, and we were open for business. Business grew briskly and I needed to expand, so I hired several sales people. Our job was to make appointments for visits to people's homes (called sits) and explain the virtues of owning land anywhere. It was the 1970's, a time in history when property was king. We would show our wonderful movie featuring Lucaya, Freeport, and Grand Bahamas in their homes and ask if they were interested in having a place in the sun to retire, or perhaps just a solid investment that would grow in value. If they weren't sure, we invited them — both husband and wife — to a dinner close to their home where we would share further details on the benefits of property ownership in the Bahamas. Then I would extend an invitation for them to come down to the island for free where we would give them a private tour of the island in a "manager's car" that was available for my use whenever I was down there.

I usually wound up going every two weeks with a new planeload of potential buyers, and I was able to take my family twice a year. It was a wonderful job and a wonderful life. The people on the island become like family to me, and I really enjoyed my interactions with the potential buyers. It felt good to help them invest in their futures. I also found that the strangest thing happens when you do something for someone else without necessarily expecting anything in return. In nine months, guess what? We were the number one office in the Real Estate Division.

We had meetings every Monday to develop the plan for the upcoming week and assist anyone who had any questions. I believed that part of the job was to see at least six people a day. Those who did would invariably see the result in above average closings. We had in-office sales contests all the time to drum up morale and friendly competition. The top performers would win fabulous dinners at great restaurants for themselves and their families if they hit a certain level of sales or saw a certain amount of prospects.

Our meetings were strong and positive, optimistic and inspiring. Everyone had to speak, whether the update for the week was good or not so good. Doing this enabled the good performers to share their tips and for not so good performers to ask for advice on how to get better. Although I don't know any one thing that made my office and staff so different than anyone else's, I do know that we surely had a winning combination that never quit.

1972 - Wantagh, New York

After a while, our family became happily entrenched in the community and we enjoyed friendships with an outstanding group of people. Business was going very well, and the kids were thriving. Steve became a talented athlete and was a star football player, as well as co-captain of both the basketball and baseball teams. He was our 3-Letter Man who hoped to become a professional football player one day. We were very proud. The twins were very popular and Larry seemed to be happy — not getting any better — but happy. Mom had adjusted well to moving back in with us after she had several minor heart attacks and Aunt Bea couldn't care for her in California anymore. I converted the garage into her own private bedroom and bath. She enjoyed helping Fritzie and I out with our busy household.

Fritzie had a job, which she seemed to enjoy for a while, and she did volunteer work at Larry's school. I thought she had gotten used to my frequent business travel, but I had this vague feeling that something was wrong even though I couldn't quite put my finger it, or I didn't want to acknowledge it. Instead, I worked even harder at my business. Before I knew it, my office became number one in all U.S. divisions. And five out of the top ten salesmen came from our office — including yours truly that took the number one spot. I asked Fritzie to please stop working, hoping that this would solve the unease that had crept into my thoughts. I assured Fritzie that we'd be fine financially and she happily agreed. She appeared excited and relieved to spend her time tending to the children, doing volunteer work and attending social engagements. But the truth of the matter was that my business success was distracting me from the fact that Fritzie was having some serious problems of her own.

To Good To Be True

Have you ever felt that things were going so well that it was too good to be true? Well, I was experiencing those feelings — and enjoying every minute of it, I might add. It seemed that we had put together "the model office" in the Perl Organization. So much so that managers from other offices were sent in to observe and told by management to incorporate what we were doing into their own operations. It is a double-edged sword when the bosses think you're great because you are highly profitable and successful, but your fellow managers hate your guts because they're getting heat for not performing as well, which is exactly what happened. Our office received accolades and I was even asked to run classes at the next convention. I had become a pretty good speaker in front of large groups, so I was told. The more you do something, the better you get. I even received the Lucaya Cup that year, which was the highest honor in the Bahama property sales division.

Things had gotten so good that we were able to build a swimming pool in the backyard of our little house in Wantagh. We had some wonderful pool parties and it felt like we were finally starting to enjoy our lives again. We'd come back from the brink and were actually able to pay off all of our bills. Including the $3000 I had borrowed from Harry Soll, my friend Bob's dad. Boy, did that feel great, and he never charged me a dime in interest. What a sweet man. I know I've said it before, but sometimes "Thank You" can't be said enough.

> **Mini-Lesson:** *Life is great if you make it great.*

Then one day, during the best week in sales that our office ever had, I received a phone call from the main office telling me to return all the money from the sales we'd made that week and start shutting down the office. We were out of business. What?!!? I truly thought that it was a prank being played on us by another office. The offices often played practical jokes and performed skits for each other to keep things fun. I thought about the last convention when our office performed a version of The Godfather for the over 2000 members of the sales organization. I played the Marlon Brando character, dressed in black with a white tie, a fedora and a toy gun, while the rest of my co-workers played my bodyguards. We did a superb job, if I do say so myself, and even got a standing "O." People talked about it for months. So naturally we assumed that another office was trying to "one-up" us.

Wrong! Until Herman Perl and Harold Blair personally got on the phone and told us that Lynden Pidling, the Prime Minister of the Bahamas, didn't want us to promote the Bahamas anymore, I didn't believe it. Apparently, Pidling wanted Bahama Realty and the Grand Bahama Development Company to close down its operations immediately. After more than eleven years, thousands of miles of roads and scores of churches, hotels, houses, golf courses, shopping bazaars, restaurants and an airport built by the Perl Organization and the Grand Bahama Development Company, they basically told us to get out of town without any notice. I had the horrible task of telling my staff of twenty that they were no longer employed. My team just couldn't comprehend how we went from having our best week ever to closing down shop overnight. But we were officially out of business. It took about a week for us to clean out our offices and for reality to set in. It was a sad time. We took the trophies we'd earned over the years home to our mantels, along with our memories of that lovely island. I still love going to the Bahamas. Only now, I am able to enjoy The Atlantis Hotel on Sol Kerzner's Paradise Island for fun in the sun. It's an incredible vacation spot with everything you need all in one location. Great job Mr. Kerzner.

Sound the Alarm

Several days later, Herman asked me to come to his office in New Jersey for a meeting. One thing about Herman was that he was never fazed by anything. He always had a plan. In fact, he always had a Plan A, B, and C. And if Plan C didn't work, he probably had a Plan D, E and F too. I had so much respect and love for him and always looked forward to being in his company. I felt smarter just being around him and tried to soak up as much as I could whenever I was in his presence. And getting a little pat on the head of appreciation from him — well, that was the greatest feeling in the world. I wish that everyone could have such a great mentor. So when I got the invitation I was relieved and nervous at the same time. I was ready for something new.

"If a man is called to be a street sweeper, he should sweep streets even as Michelangelo painted or Beethoven composed music, or Shakespeare wrote poetry. He should sweep streets so well that all the hosts of heaven and earth will pause to say: Here lived a great street sweeper who did his job well."
— Martin Luther King, Jr.

When I arrived at Herman's office he told me that because I had done so well selling real estate, he wanted to offer me a new opportunity in another area of the organization. He asked if I was interested in learning the burglar and fire alarm business. He had an open spot in New Jersey for a few months to educate me on all aspects of the security business, and then there would be a chance for me to manage the Connecticut office of Dictograph Security Systems, eventually perhaps even becoming a franchisee. I was a bit shocked for a moment. I knew nothing about the security business, except that it was a much harder sale because you're selling the homeowner on his or her fears, as opposed to their hopes, which is what I had been selling in the real estate biz. My first question was how long the training would take, as I wasn't technically inclined at all. Then I inquired how much the top guns in the business made, as I heard that it was a fairly low-paying business, with long hours and a lot of evening appointments.

Herman responded, "What you've heard about the business is true. However, there is an evolution going on right now, and people's needs for protection of their property, equipment and even their lives are changing. The way the business has been run in the past is not going to work anymore, and I need you to help lead the change. Nothing is more constant than change, Walter. Don't forget that." (I never did). Wow, was I flattered. No one could challenge Herman's success and good fortune, and if he believed in me, that was saying a lot. And although I didn't know the security business, by now what I did know was that I could sell. And just as I had learned to run the salons, car wash and real estate businesses, I figured I could learn the security business, too. So, I accepted. I called Fritzie at home and said, "Guess what, honey, we're in a new business — home security." She replied, "I knew you would join Mr. Perl in anything. I'm happy for you and for us."

I soon started working in the New Jersey office and felt like a little kid back in school again. In many ways I was. Learning a whole new business and getting exposure to a new group of great teachers was invigorating, and as always, I was eager to learn. I am particularly thankful for the lessons that Mr. Mitch Resnick taught me. Mitch, who was known as "The Train," worked his way up through the ranks of the security business to become the president of the franchise organization. He was a perpetually positive man who truly believed that his mission was to save lives and help people by providing them with the security protection they needed. He made a huge impact on me and we became close. He even gave me a copy of *As a Man Thinketh* by James Allen, which Mitch inscribed for me with the message "To Walter, My brother in-heart." The book, written in 1902, essentially talks about the power of our thoughts. I still have it and it's something that I will always hold dear to my heart. Thanks Mitch, for the support, guidance and friendship.

> **Mini-Lesson:** *Always continue to keep building relationships that are real and meaningful.*

I also got the chance to work with a gentleman by the name of Jim Wyler. Working with Jim reminded me of being in the Army again. He was that regimented. He was a vitamin junkie and followed the exact same routine every day, including working out. Before long he got me to join him, and I credit him for getting me back in pretty good shape. Jim was a force of nature and was capable of doing it all. He ran his own numbers and wrote his own sales programs. He did for Dictograph Security what had never been done there before and would be hard to repeat today. His philosophy was that any salesman should see at least two people per day, or 40 per month, and if they knew their stuff, they would sell 25% of them. It was a set program that Jim strictly followed and firmly believed in.

I decided to take it a step further and see at least six people per day, or 120 per month, and sell at least 40% of them, to be even further ahead that way. Jim was doubtful that it could be done, but I did just that. He loved it and loved me for it. Working with Jim inspired me and strengthened my already strong work ethic by showing me that there was a degree of science to sales. It was a numbers game. The more people you see, the more you sell — as long as you know what you are talking about and believe in what you are selling. If you truly believe that you are providing a helpful product or service to your customer, that is a very powerful proposition. I have always been a firm believer and continually try to take it a step further.

When the long daily commute from Long Island to Florham Park, NJ became problematic, Herman got a two bedroom apartment nearby for Jim and I to share during the week. Sometimes when we needed some time alone, I'd bring Fritzie to the apartment on the weekend and we'd leave my mother in charge of the children. Fritzie would sometimes help me send out brochures and letters to prospective buyers as part of our sales program.

After about three months of learning the business, I still hadn't made a sale (or a commission) and I was getting a little anxious. I began to question myself and wondered if I could be the salesman and manager that I was before. It's easy to walk on water when you know where the rocks are, but then I started to think bigger, and I had an idea. Why just focus on individual homeowners? So I began to target larger entities — insurance companies, realtors and the like. I drove to Englewood, New Jersey, near the George Washington Bridge and went into a few places to practice my sales technique. I dutifully rehearsed my presentation in the car prior to going into each new place. I was out there alone, selling, and the excitement started to get my juices flowing. I truly believed that I was doing something very real — potentially saving someone's life. That became my main focus and motivation.

It's been said in some of the circles, that if you took away the power, prestige, and money from winners, some of them — the true believers and hard workers — would be right back where they were, or even better in a short period of time. I've always believed if you want to find out if you're a true competitor in the sales world, you should fly to any city with another sales rep. You both have a credit card for gas, $500 in cash and a suitcase of clothes. No product. Just you, your imagination and your sales skills. At the end of 30 days, you meet again, and assess how well you both did. Whoever has the most money, wins. I never tried it, but I've thought about it often and someday, would love to, just for fun.

Anyway, I went into a real estate office not expecting much. I hoped at the very least that they'd give me a list of new homeowners in the area. Then it happened — I got my break. I walked in, introduced myself and almost hit the floor when the owner said, "Come in. I need to talk to you." He looked me straight in the eye and asked me if I really knew my business. I told him I was as close to an expert as he could get (talk about a positive attitude). He explained that he was having a problem with his insurance company. They were requiring him to immediately install a fire alarm system in a small apartment building that he owned in order to keep his coverage. He gave me the address of the building and I told him I'd get him an estimate as soon as possible. So I drove about two miles to the four-story walk-up. But when I knocked on the doors to get an idea of the scope of the job, no one was home.

Although I wasn't able to get in to see any of the apartments, I'd been told they were all one bedrooms with the same layout. I was alone, so I made an executive decision. I filled out the estimate: one heat detector and two smoke detectors in front of each apartment, one in each apartment, and an outside alarm with a control panel in the attic. I drove back to the owner about one hour later. Shocked to see me back so soon, he said, "That's some service." I told him how important it was to me to do a good job and service my clients promptly. He was impressed. I wrote up my first order for $3000 and asked for a 50% deposit. He signed the papers, gave me a check and asked when the installation would happen. "Almost immediately," I said. I thanked him for his business, he thanked me for my quick service, we shook hands and I was off and running into my newest career. In fact, I drove right back to Florham Park at about 75 miles an hour to share the news.

I walked around like a peacock with full feathers until Herman and Jim saw my contract. They laughed for weeks and never let me forget the description on my alarm installation that simply read, "17, just spread them out." I assumed that the installers would know where to place the equipment, but it was company policy that the salesman not only list the quantity needed, but put every placement down in the contract in exact, itemized detail. Oh well, live and learn, right? Even though they got a kick out of my contract, they were proud of me, and I was proud of myself. I never did quite live down the "17, spread 'em out Levine" label, but it was my first big sale and I was thrilled.

Herman sent out Pete Pugliese, his main installer, to check the job and see where everything should go. I found out that I didn't plan for enough heat and smoke detectors in the building in order for it to be adequately protected. But Herman accepted the job at the $3000 price and made up the difference of $700 in the additional equipment needed out of his own pocket. He covered everything, and he never charged me back. Herman Perl was a great man who never ceased to amaze me with his generosity and kind, caring nature. I think he enjoyed seeing me, a novice in the business, with minimal knowledge, come back with a big sale and a big smile, and he didn't want to take the wind out of my sails. He was a great motivator and mentor.

> **Mini-Lesson:** *If your business isn't moving fast enough consider the turtle, it can't move at all if it doesn't stick his neck out. You can't make it happen if you're not persistent. Go out, shake hands and make new friends.*

After that, I went back to my new friend and client in the real estate office and asked for referrals, which he was happy to give me. It wasn't long before I started to write business in New Jersey on a daily basis, and I started feeling like a champion again, enjoying every moment. Jim was recruiting his former lieutenants from the real estate business, and it seemed we always had someone sleeping in the living room of the apartment.

It was getting crowded in the apartment, and I knew that six months of training was more than enough for me. Herman knew it, too. He called me in and said to me, "You're ready. I have a franchise I'm terminating in Norwalk, Connecticut, owned by a Fairfield County family. They did not meet my needs in Connecticut, so here's $10,000 in your account. Get a secretary, an office, some furniture and interview the three guys that worked for the old franchise to see if you want them to work for you." It was "déjà vu all over again." My body was tingling. What a great feeling.

> **Mini-Lesson:** *Anyone who thinks he or she is indispensible should stick a finger in a bowl of water and notice how long the hole stays after your finger is pulled out. To improve your odds at success, be the first one in and the last one out.*

1974 - Wantagh, New York

In world news at the time, Richard Nixon had resigned from the Presidency after the scandal of the Watergate break-in, and Gerald Ford stepped up to take over the job as leader of the free world. In our little corner of the world, my family was excited about moving to Connecticut, or at least I thought they were. The truth was, only Fritzie and I were. In fact, after taking a few rides to Connecticut from Long Island, Fritzie loved it and could hardly wait. She hoped that it might be our final move.

Steve asked if he could finish his final year of high school in Wantagh, where he'd become a football hero. And the girls, Leslie and Lori, who were still very much into cheerleading and gymnastics, didn't want to lose their friends. Fritzie and I decided to wait to make the move. It was not the right time and it was more important right now for the children to be happy. I had to tolerate the long commute from Wantagh to Norwalk and back each day. Almost 2 hours each way. It was a lot of wear and tear on both the car and on me.

> **Mini-Lesson:** *Love yourself enough to make a difference in your own life, even if it will affect those you love. There are no guarantees in life. No, you don't know how (or if) it's going to work out. But for your sake as well as theirs, you must try.*

So I opened the office in Norwalk on the second floor of an unassuming two-story building at 69 East Avenue above an insurance office. I put ads in the local papers for a secretary, but convinced Judy Trupin, my childhood friend to take the job. I also interviewed the three salesmen who had worked for the previous franchisee. I asked them if they wanted to work with me. They all seemed knowledgeable and very personable, and they agreed to come on board.

I told them my sales philosophy of trying to help the customer and then told them we would split the territories, one person per community. I asked them to each pick an area they wanted to focus on. One chose New Canaan and Darien, stating they were wealthy communities that he was intimately familiar with. Another chose Fairfield and Westport. When I asked him why, he said that it was close to his home, and he knew a lot of people in the area. The third man chose Stamford — saying that it was a big city with a large population, and he'd really be able to build a business out of the community. I questioned why not one of them had chosen Greenwich, the wealthiest town in the entire state. They said that they'd all worked that area at some point, but there were now over 130 alarm companies listed in the Greenwich Yellow Pages, so it was not likely that there were many alarm systems left to be installed there.

I didn't know enough about either the business, the area or the market need, but I was thinking about the question of *"How Can I Help You?"* and I wanted to put some of my sales theories into action, so I said that I would work Greenwich. It was on my route to and from the office and I welcomed the challenge. I would stop each way and see if I could find some business and build my name and reputation. Greenwich has many magnificent homes, both old and new, with some of the older ones built by the Rockefellers, Winthrops, Otis Elevator heirs, Victor Borge and others — you get the idea.

> **Mini-Lesson:** *I knew I had to introduce myself to all that would listen. Operating a business without advertising is like winking at a beautiful woman in the dark — you know what you're doing, but no one else does.*

I couldn't understand why these three seemingly smart, ambitious salesmen would avoid the wealthiest town in the entire state, where so many other companies had thought to set up operations. I believed that there was still gold to be had in them there hills. And, as it turned out, boy, was I right! The first thing I did was to introduce myself to the Chief of Police and the Fire Chief, a tactic learned from good old Jerry the Tin Man. I guess I did learn something from the guy, after all. Although, luckily, I never followed in his questionable "bait and switch" footsteps. The chiefs wound up introducing me to a lot of great people on both forces, which led to some helpful connections, but in the meantime, I needed business — now.

The first house I knocked on the door of was a home in a beautiful section of Greenwich called Deer Park. A man opened the door, listened to me while I did my presentation, and when I was finished, he said, "Walter, by your own admission there are 130 alarm companies in the Greenwich Yellow Pages. Why should I buy from you?" I thought for a moment, and then answered honestly, "Well, you would be my only customer. Just think what great service you'll get!" He chuckled, shook his head and said that he couldn't argue with that. Then he wrote me a check and signed a contract on the spot. At the time, I didn't realize who exactly my first customer was, but I came to find out that his name was David Wallace, Chairman of Bunga Punta Corporation, owners of Smith & Wesson, Cessna and many other companies. I'll always be thankful that he and his wife took a chance on me and gave my business its start in Greenwich. After that, it was like my birthday every day. There was business everywhere and the nicest people (mostly) to meet and greet — and of course, sell.

> **Mini-Lesson:** *Opportunity knocks again. Remember the door is wide open! Another person's program or system that is not working is an opportunity for you — but only if you recognize it and do something about it.*

I started to build up a very good reputation with some wonderful clients who really believed in and came to depend on me. A large part of the clientele I developed included some large and isolated houses in the "back country" of Greenwich. I would often drive out there to check in on or service my accounts, and found that you need to use the bathroom while you're out there in the middle of nowhere, it pays to have a few friends in the area. I had about five very nice people who always welcomed a "stop-over" from me at their houses for cookies and a bathroom break.

One of them was a little old lady who was always very nice to me. She was very wealthy (her late husband founded a world renowned food company) and also very sheltered. One day after one of my stop-overs, she asked me to do her a favor. "Of course," I said. "What is it?" "See what happens when you let one in?" she muttered angrily as we walked toward the door. I asked her what she was talking about and why she was so upset. She said, "I don't mean you. You're different." I suddenly realized that she was referring to the fact that I was Jewish. Then she continued, "Someone bought the house and now has two separate families living there. Could you imagine? Can you please go down the street and check things out? It's the house with two names on the mailbox."

I said that was hard to believe, especially considering the neighborhood. Although I honestly didn't understand why it would bother her so much. I guess I didn't have the same level of outrage partly because I didn't live there, but also because I had been brought up to always take care of family, and if necessary, that could include extended family living with you. But happy to oblige, I went down the road to check things out. Sure enough, there were in fact two listings on the mailbox. One was obviously a Jewish family name, but the other read "Gan Eden," which perplexed me.

Without a second thought, I knocked on the door and a lovely lady answered. I told her one of the neighbors mentioned that she had just bought the house and thought she might need a burglar and fire alarm system. She said, as a matter of fact, she did need one and we proceeded to survey the house together so that I could write up an estimate. She mentioned that she'd heard her new neighbors speak of me in high regard, so she trusted me with her business. I was pleased to hear that I had such a good reputation with my clients.

When we were finished touring the home, I got up the nerve to ask her where the other family lived. "What other family?" she asked. When I mentioned the two names on the mailbox, she laughed out loud and said, "Walter, I thought you were Jewish?" I assured her that I was, and

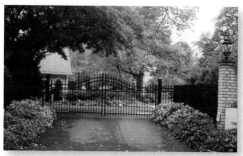

Entrance to Walter's Beachside Avenue home, Westport, CT.

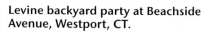

Levine backyard party at Beachside Avenue, Westport, CT.

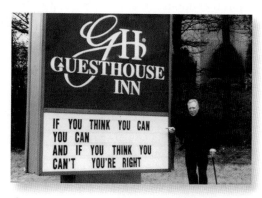

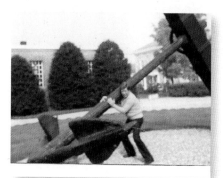

Walter's had a lot of "heavy things" to carry around in his life.

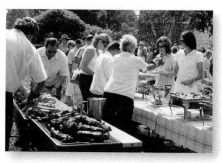

IF YOU THINK YOU CAN
YOU CAN
AND IF YOU THINK YOU
CAN'T YOU'RE RIGHT

The sign on the marquee honoring Walter's arrival with one of his many motivational quotes, at the Guesthouse Inn (where he stayed during his cancer treatments) in Little Rock, AR.

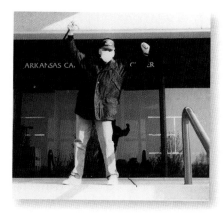

Leaving the Arkansas Research Center triumphantly, after completing treatment (1992).

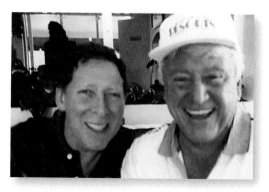

Walter and Merv Griffin at the Paradise Island Hotel in the Bahamas, Nassau (1994).

All photos courtesy of M. Walter Levine

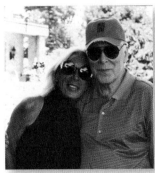

Judy Trupin, one of Walter's dearest childhood friends, with Walter at the Beachside home in Westport, CT.

Joel Gutterman (a.k.a "1A"— he and Walter grew up in same apartment building in Brooklyn) giving a toast at Walter's 50th birthday party, as Bob Soll (another childhood friend), Fritzie, Walter and a member of the band look on. Bluewater Hill house in Westport, CT (January, 1987).

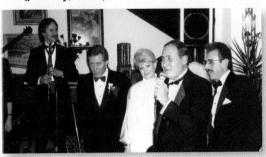

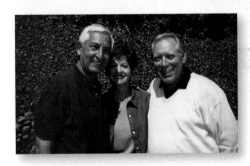

Walter with cousin Ira and Barbara Fine. Ira and Walter have been like brothers from different mothers for most of their lives.

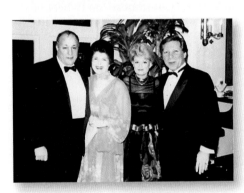

Herb and Helen Gordon at Walter's 50th birthday party. Herb introduced Walter to the sea cucumber (TBL-12) supplement, which Walter takes daily for his health and to prevent cancer reoccurrence.

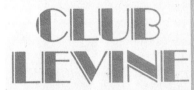

An invitation to one of the many parties the Levines hosted at their home in Westport, CT.

All photos courtesy of M. Walter Levine

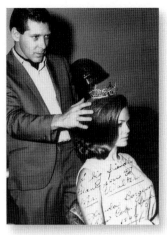

Doing the hair of Linda Borgenson for the Miss America contest at his Colorado salon (1966).

Walter's Revlon days – doing a makeup presentation on Miss Uruguay from the Miss Universe pageant at Burdine's Department Store.

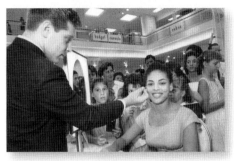

A family stroll in New York, while taking the kids to see the Statue of Liberty (1966).

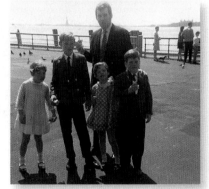

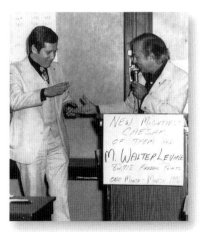

Walter receiving a Piaget watch from mentor, Herman Perl, for winning the "Mightiest Caesar of them All" award.

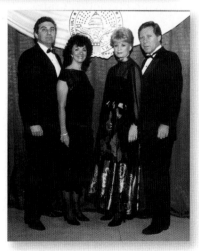

Fritzie and Walter at the Ronald Reagan and George H.W. Bush Inaugural Ball with their friends (January 1985).

All photos courtesy of M. Walter Levine

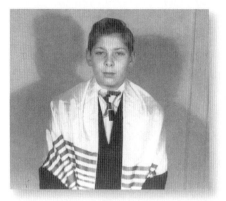

Walter on the day of his Bar Mitzvah (January 14, 1950).

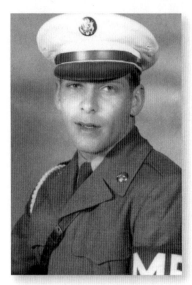

Walter at 18 years old, while in the U.S. Miliary Police, Augusta, Georgia (1955).

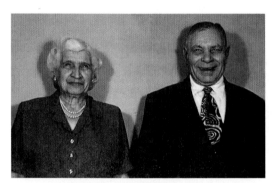

Bub and Pop (1949) — Walter's grandparents (on his mother's side).

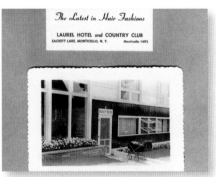

Walter's first beauty salon at the Laurel Hotel & Country Club in the Catskill Mountains (1960). Baby Steve's carriage stands outside.

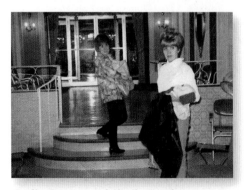

Eydie Gorme and Sheila Kershner leaving the Concord Hotel Salon after getting their hair done (January 1966).

All photos courtesy of M. Walter Levine

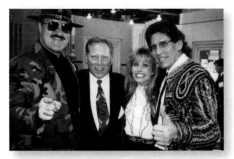

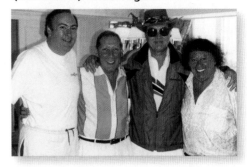

David Fishoff (sports & entertainment agent), Walter, Steve Rossi and Marty Allen (comedians) in Las Vegas.

Sgt. Slaughter, Walter, Debbie Fields (of Mrs. Fields' Cookies) and Tito Santana at the Las Vegas Television Convention, during Walter's stint as a wrestling manager.

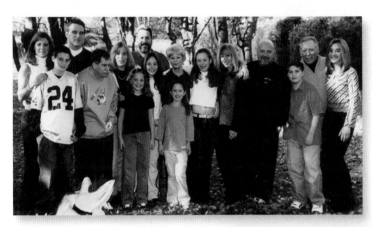

Walter and his family outside the front of his Beachside Avenue home in Westport, CT (2000).

Taking the grandkids out for a ride in the Rolls Royce Walter bought after he was told he had just days to live (1996).

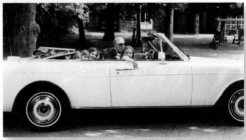

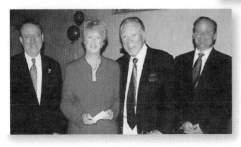

Peter Omera and Connecticut Governor Jodi Rell, with Walter and his friend and attorney Gabe Selig at a dinner recognizing Walter's fundraising efforts for children's charities (2002).

All photos courtesy of M. Walter Levine

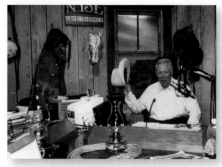

Walter at the Imus Ranch, sitting behind Don Imus' desk (2002).

Carl Ruderman (Owner & Publisher of Elite Traveler Magazine), Geraldine Ferrara (politician), Richard Grasso (former CEO of New York Stock Exchange), John McCain (politician), Fritzie and Walter at a prostate cancer fundraiser in NYC (2004).

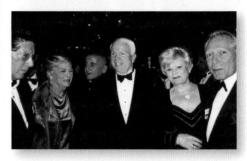

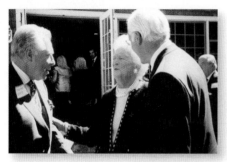

Walter meeting Barbara Bush at a fundraiser (2007).

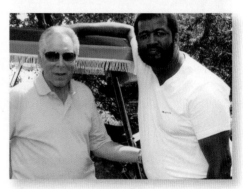

Long-time employee and "other son," Leroy. Walter doesn't know what he'd do without him.

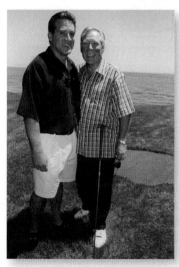

Walter and son Steve hitting some golf balls at Beachside Avenue home.

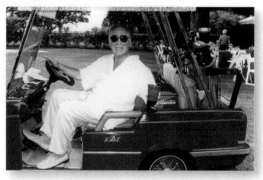

The "$4 million dollar golf-cart" Walter got from a former golf executive and client who paid Walter his share of a settlement with it. He had his son Larrry's initials engraved on the door.

All photos courtesy of M. Walter Levine

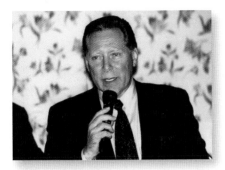

Walter giving one of his inspiring motivational speeches.

Visiting the old neighborhood — East Flatbush, Brooklyn. The former apartment building where Walter grew up and started his first business (selling clothespins to the ladies) is now a parking lot, laced in barbed wire.

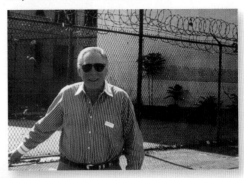

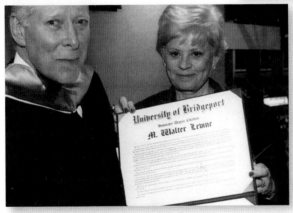

Fritzie giving Walter smiles on receiving his Honorary Doctorate (2004).

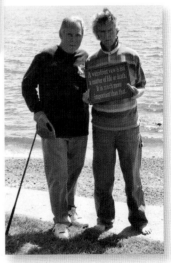

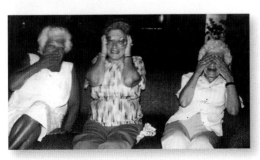

The Butler Sisters — Walter's mom, Fay, with his Aunt Syd and Aunt Bea doing their "See no evil, hear no evil, speak no evil," routine (yeah, right!!).

Walter and Imus hangin out by the sound in Walter's backyard in Westport, CT.

All photos courtesy of M. Walter Levine

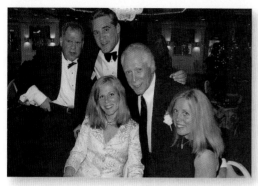

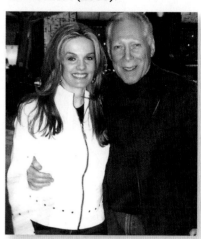

Walter and Diana at a casino in Connecticut (2008).

Larry, Steve, Walter, Lori and Leslie at the Fritzie Levine Gala Celebration given by the State of CT (2009).

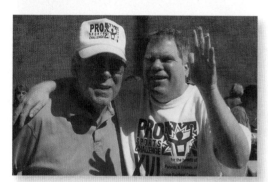

Walter with son Larry at the Pro Sports Challenge to benefit the Lower Fairfield Center (1998).

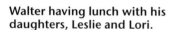

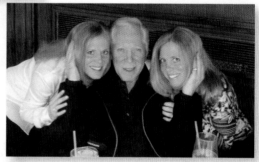

Walter having lunch with his daughters, Leslie and Lori.

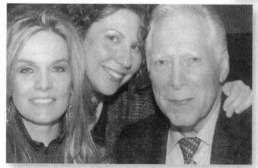

Diana, Virginia Juliano (this book's co-author) and Walter.

All photos courtesy of M. Walter Levine

then she proceeded to explain to me that "Gan Eden" meant "the Garden of Eden" in Hebrew and was the name she and her husband gave their home. Feeling a bit like a schmuck, I explained that I did go to Hebrew School, but that I wasn't a very good student.

We had a good laugh about it, and I got the order. Years later when Fritzie and I built our dream home on the water in Westport, Connecticut, I knew exactly what I wanted to name it. "Gan Eden," of course. We hoped it would be our sanctuary for many years to come, and in many ways it was. I don't remember the last name of the sweet Jewish woman I met that day, but the name of her home and what it stood for stayed with me long after. I especially remember how she made me feel and how she opened up the possibility of having a Garden of Eden of my own some day.

> **Mini-Lesson:** *Think and live each day better than yesterday. Live for the future. What you learned yesterday is the vision that builds your dreams of tomorrow.*

Walter's ABCDs

One day, I asked a client of mine for the name of his insurance broker. That's how I came to meet a great guy by the name of Don Cleveland. Don had been a broker in Greenwich for 70 years. I showed up at our first appointment with a cup of coffee for him and a cup of tea for me, and told him that I really wanted to understand the insurance business better. Don gave me his download, and he also told me about a man who he was friends with named Percy Chubb, the owner of an insurance company bearing his name. He told me that he would be helpful to speak with and gave me his number. What happened next was not only history, but it would cement my ideas regarding the power of timing and tenacity. I called Mr. Chubb's New York office several times.

His staff was very nice, but they repeatedly told me that he'd call me back, to no avail. Two months went by as I regularly attempted to reach him through his office. Finally, I asked Herman Perl if he knew Percy Chubb, and Herman did indeed know him — they both lived in the suburban town of Short Hills, New Jersey. I asked Herman if I could use his name and for Mr. Chubb's street address, because I wanted to make a house call. Herman thought I was crazy, but he gave me the man's address and the okay to use his name. Early one evening, I drove to Mr. Chubb's house and knocked on his door at about 7:00 p.m. He answered the door himself, and I told him my name and mentioned that Herman Perl was my mentor and friend. I said, "Mr. Perl says you're a very nice man. I've tried to reach you at your New York office for two months, so I asked Mr. Perl for your address and drove here from Norwalk, Connecticut. May I please have just two minutes of your time?"

> **Mini-Lesson:** *You gotta take chances if it feels right.*

He asked me if I was crazy. I said, "I have an idea which can save your company millions of dollars." He paused, looked at his watch, and then said, "You know Herman Perl? Okay, you've got two minutes. Come on in." When we were seated in his living room, I continued, "If you offered a discount to homeowners who own art, jewelry, cash and other valuables in their homes and offices if they had a security and fire alarm system approved by your company, you'd probably save a lot of money on payouts for burglaries and fires, wouldn't you?" Mr. Chubb smiled and said, "You drove all the way here from Connecticut just to ask me that question?"

He then inquired as to where I was going from there, and I told him I was driving right back to Connecticut. He asked if I'd eaten dinner, and I told him that I had not. With that, Percy Chubb asked his wife to please put out another plate at the table, and I was asked to stay for dinner. We discussed my idea, which he liked very much, and when I left, he asked for my business card and said someone would be in touch with me. The next week, I received twelve calls to set up appointments with Chubb Insurance Company clients. Before I knew what was happening, dozens of insurance company brokers were phoning me asking for surveys and installations for homes in and around Greenwich, Stamford and Westchester County, New York.

It took me to a whole new level within the security business. Percy Chubb and I had discussed a 10% discount, and it worked out nicely for all of the insurers at the time. Nowadays, insurance companies offer 20% or more off their rates to clients with security systems, which makes me smile in satisfaction. To think that perhaps an idea of mine made a difference and saved a lot of people a lot of money, makes me very proud. Herman was very proud of me then too. He honored me with a Piaget watch with the inscription, "To Walter Levine, who aims and hits the sky — March 1976." It was the last gift I ever received from him, though certainly not the first. He gave me the gift of his belief in me and shared his enthusiasm and business knowledge. He was truly a mentor and friend. Around that time I was also awarded the first Herman Perl Sales Award called, "Applause from Salesmen Everywhere." I still have it in my office. It's a sculpture of clapping hands that Herman created especially for me. He dabbled in sculpting as a hobby, and it's something that I still cherish.

> **Mini-Lesson:** *Doing the right thing is always more important than doing things right. Luck is what happens when persistence meets opportunity.*

From that point on, it was incredible. I became the number one salesperson in the company, and five out of the top ten salesmen in the Perl Organization came from my office. All of the accolades in the world were bestowed upon me. This was really happening! As you can imagine, that's something most of us can never get enough of. Nobody could understand what we were doing in our little office in Norwalk, but they couldn't deny that it was successful. We started getting visitors from the other offices throughout the country to find out what our magic formula was. It made me realize that in order to sustain and scale our success, we needed to formalize the techniques we were using and give it a name that conveyed the larger concept of what we were doing. That's when I came up with the "ABDCs of Selling and of Life." Not only did it tell the story of our belief in what we were doing — selling our systems that protected lives and property — but it was also catchy and easy to remember. In my opinion, our success all boiled down to 4 points — Attitude, Believability, Commitment and Discipline.

"If you tried to do something but couldn't, you are better off than if you had tried to do nothing and succeeded."
— John T. Ragland, Jr.

In my opinion attitude is the foundation for all of your life. With a positive attitude, you could take on the world. Without it, you're toast. Believability is getting your customer's trust. But the only way to get that is to truly know your stuff. Sure, sometimes one has to punt during the sales process, but if you have a strong basis of knowledge, you can honestly admit the few times when you don't know the answer, without feeling like a failure, but assure them that you'll find out and get back to them, and most importantly, you'd better follow up and make sure you do it.

That brings us to the next one, Commitment. You must be 1000% committed to reaching your goal. Nothing, and I mean nothing, will stand in your way. You can give it lip service, but unless you follow through, you'll only go so far. That leads us to Discipline. You need to have a regimen or routine that reinforces your commitment and goals. Making 6 sales calls every day, no matter what. Rehearsing before every presentation, without fail. "Sales" is certainly an art form, but Discipline allows you to create more of a science out of sales, which in turn creates more consistent results, and that guarantees success.

> **Mini-Lesson:** *Think positive and keep smiling. Every day is a new day. Knowledge is a light – don't forget to turn it on daily.*

We had a dedicated team that focused on these four points relentlessly. I stressed them over and over and never let up. We would not accept anything short of success and our team became laser focused on the ABCDs. I began to have mandatory meetings every Friday morning at 8:45am, instead of on Mondays. Be on time, or don't come to work. We had a near-perfect attendance at all of our meetings, We would serve bagels, cream cheese, juice, and coffee and I was told that the fever pitch in the room was similar to that of a preacher with his flock. I guess I felt a true urgency to pass on my beliefs, and you can bet I did. Busloads of salesmen from Washington, DC, Maryland, Allentown, PA, and even people from Washington state came to see what we were doing differently. People were moving outside of their comfort zone, and finding that the journey became an adventure.

During our many conventions across the country I was challenged by many of my peers. They would tell me that they were going to surpass my achievements and beat my sales the following year. There was an annual sales contest with everyone starting evenly. Each year, I accepted the challenges and enjoyed the rivalry and banter between the offices and the salespeople. The phone calls were hot and heavy for about three or four months with many of us in a dead heat, but then they started dropping like flies. I guess they had a bad month or two and just gave up, thinking it was all over.

It's okay to have a bad day, week or even month, as long as you believe that it will change. You don't know if it's luck of the draw, something personal that took your attention away or maybe you just couldn't keep up the pace. Whatever. It's okay. The trick is to know that your dry spell will end sometime, if you let it. In fact, you can help it end sooner by slowing down. Stop, look around, think positively, use your imagination and visualize. Believe that whomever you are going to see needs you and they can't say no to something they need and want. I guarantee that you will receive the order, and you will feel better because your goal will seem all the more reachable. Find your passion and fear not.

It was sometimes difficult to help some of my challengers to their feet. I tried to help them anyway, despite their fears of losing, feeling uncomfortable and losing face, but many just walked away. Why would I want to help them, you ask? Because it's lonely at the top! The truth is, if you ask any winner whom he or she enjoys sharing their success with, you'll probably hear that sharing it with another winner is up there at the top. It's a terrific feeling. That's probably the reason why I love charity work and get true satisfaction from helping someone out. It's pure magic for me. It's also another reason why I help cancer patients and their families, because nothing makes me feel as good as helping them; giving them the "hope" that they need to beat cancer, as I did, is indescribably gratifying.

> **Mini-Lesson:** *The road to success is always under construction. It is never over, but you must continually visualize success in order to make it to your destination.*

Before long, our office's sales programs became the company standard because no one could deny that they worked. And our sales record continued to be the best in the company. It was truly a career high point. I remembered those words of good old Jay Levan, and I certainly took them to heart. In order to be number one you need to do more than everyone else — see more people than anybody else, rehearse more, truly want to help people, and ask the important questions, including the most important one: *"How Can I Help You?"* Listen carefully for the answers, find out what people really need and try to help them get it. It's quite easy to do the right thing. I was able to pass on to my team my passion for success and doing well. Attitude is the key to building just about everything and beating anything. It will make you strong enough to believe you can beat the odds and reach success. I'd always known that I was not an intellectually educated man, but I always believed that I made up for it with street smarts, pride, righteousness and drive.

> **Mini-Lesson:** *The mind is the most powerful tool you have. Your mind conceives what your heart believes. Happiness and being great at what you do are directly related to knowing how to do your job well and your attitude about it.*

As a salesman, most of the time I was able to determine within the first few minutes if I was accepted or rejected by a potential new client. I tried to never waste time selling something to someone who was not at all interested in my product. Sometimes my all-important question *"How Can I Help You?"* fell on deaf ears. I would get answers like "Thank you, but I don't need your help," or even "Get lost!" At least I knew where I stood. What's even worse is the "Let me think about it." Or the "Call me in a week or two." Or "I'll get back to you." Any vague "maybe" without honesty is such a waste of time for a salesman, and will literally put you out of business. In my opinion, a quick "No thank you" is better than fruitlessly pursuing a sale when you really don't have a chance.

As I became more successful, I was invited into the homes and lives of even more successful people. I loved every moment of it and looked at each encounter as a learning opportunity. Doctors, businessmen, professional athletes and the like all thought enough of me to invite me to their tables and break bread with their families. I'd like to thank you all again for making me a part of your family and your lives. It was an experience and an education that I'll never forget.

> **Mini-Lesson:** *Business is like riding a bicycle. Either you keep up your speed or you're going to fall down.*

The Gold Coast

One night, I went to dinner at Judy Trupin's. My old friend had built a beautiful new house in Westport, Connecticut. During the course of conversation, I mentioned that the commute from Wantagh to Norwalk was really getting to me. I complained about having to wake up at 5:30 a.m. to make early morning appointments in Greenwich and the late rides home every night at 10 p.m. or later. Sweet Judy invited me to live with her family for as long as I needed to, for two or three nights a week, though I'd have to share a bathroom with their daughter Tara. Tara was the same age as my twin girls, so I came to think of her as another daughter of mine. She was a good sport and didn't complain much. Tara the trooper put up with my one-hour bathroom routine, which was my only free time. It lasted seventeen months before Barry, Judy's husband finally said, "Walter, I love ya, but enough is enough. Get out!" I was the man who came to dinner and stayed for a year and a half. How many people would put up with that? Not many. Thank you, Judy. You are a saint and I love you like a sister. You are my sister.

Mini-Lesson: *Reducing my time on the road increased my sales and the sales of my team. Being close to your working family can be a very beneficial thing.*

During that time, I was going home to Long Island on Wednesday and Friday nights and on weekends. I often had to drive back and forth on Saturdays and some Sundays because that was the only time potential clients could meet with me. I took Steve with me when I could to teach him the world of sales. My team continued to break records for new installations and I was making more money than I ever had before in my life — somewhere between $80,000 and $100,000 a year. It was big money to me at the time.

Fritzie and I finally decided that it was time to make the move to Connecticut. We put our house in Wantagh up for sale and bought a big house in Trumbull, Connecticut. It was over 3500 square feet in size, three levels on a corner lot, and over an acre of property. We began the move and decorating process, and I was fortunate to have a client in Greenwich in the furniture business who helped us with all the furniture we needed. Although we were thrilled about our move to the Gold Coast (as the Fairfield County area is known, due to its large concentration of wealth), the kids were still not happy about the prospect at all.

The move took its toll on the whole family, and this period of time was very rough emotionally for all of us. Steve was planning to leave for Villanova University in Pennsylvania, and Leslie and Lori were now fourteen and in high school. It isn't easy making new friends and giving up all that you know, especially at that age. It's a tough time of life to begin with, and trying to fit into a new social world at a new school made it even harder, but everyone adjusted over time. We all got through it as a family, and eventually all of the kids couldn't imagine living anywhere else. Today, they've all made wonderful lives for themselves and their families in Connecticut, with lifelong friends and deep ties to the community.

The next important thing on the agenda was Larry. At this point he was a teenager, and we knew he needed to be with other kids like him — he needed friends. We focused on getting him into a local program so he wouldn't be too far away from us. I'd heard about a new building and program in Norwalk which had opened the year before. It was called the Lower Fairfield Regional Center, and when we went to look at the facility and we absolutely loved it. Unfortunately, they told us it was full, but they would put us on the waiting list. I really fell in love with the place, and went back three or four times, basically begging to get Larry in. I called one of my former clients in Long Island, who travelled in political circles, for advice. They directed me to the great lady named Mary Anne Crupsick, who was the Lieutenant Governor of New York at the time.

Turns out I had met her before when she spent some time working the Nassau County Retarded Children Association, and she was very gracious. Before I knew it, she was on the phone to the Governor of Connecticut, Ella Grasso, telling her what a great find it would be to have Fritzie and Walter Levine on the team to help raise money and work for the benefit of all the kids in the state that needed help with mental retardation. The very next day, we received a call from the Lower Fairfield Regional Center telling us to bring Larry, as well as his clothes and personal belongings there, as they were able to secure space for him. We were ecstatically happy, yet sad at the same time, and we couldn't stop crying. Larry, for the first time in his life, would have a real connection to other people he could relate to other than his family. In fact, the other people at the center would soon become his new family of friends. The staff was incredible, and still is to this day. I must also mention the professionalism of the Governor, Commissioner, Lt. Commissioner, the State Staff, and all of the people that really "get it." They have developed a wonderful program of caring for people who need it the most. They are like Larry's second family. Thank you from the bottom of our hearts for making the dream of a good life for our son a total reality. He adapted quickly to his new surroundings and loved it almost immediately. We still bring Larry home every Sunday with the family. It's known in our family as "Sundays with Larry." Sound familiar?

> **Mini-Lesson:** *Good things come to those who wait, as long as they work like hell while they wait.*

Fritzie and I followed through with our promise of supporting the Center, and started a group called the Parents and Friends of Lower Fairfield Regional Center. Fritzie was co-president with a great lady named Cindy Stromandinoli. Fritzie and Cindy became best friends, and we spent a lot of time with her and her husband, Dom, who was a fantastic guy as well. Cindy and Dom had two children in the facility and they were as equally committed as Fritzie and I to making it the best place that it could be. Both ladies made themselves known throughout the State of Connecticut as committed advocates appointed for the LFCRC (Lower Fairfield County Regional Center). They became like sisters, driving to Hartford, the state capitol, for critical votes and meetings with politicians, even though only one of them was needed. That's love and sisterhood.

> **Mini-Lesson:** *Develop friendships that earn one another's respect. You wind up making a life-long friend and family member on the same team, with the benefit of doing good for all.*

The End of an Era

In May of 1976, as the nation was preparing to celebrate the Bicentennial of our country, a 53-year-old Herman Perl had a massive, fatal stroke in his office in Florham Park, New Jersey. I had just been to see him there two weeks earlier to pick up a beautiful, inscribed Piaget watch that he bought for me. His gift and gesture was meant to recognize my sales performance and encourage others to follow my example. It meant the world to me. When I got the news of his death, I was absolutely devastated. I basically went from the highest point in my life to the deepest level of sadness overnight. At the funeral, all of Herman's friends, family and business associates came together and cried for the loss of a great friend, advisor, and for me, father figure. Herman was my surrogate father and treated me like a son more times than I could've possibly deserved. Herman Perl was a true champion. A top-notch salesman with the vision and discipline to see things through. He was also a warm-hearted individual who enjoyed helping others. His influence on me was enormous and I will always miss him and be thankful for having had him in my life.

> **Mini-Lesson:** *If you have the opportunity to mentor someone and help them develop a career or a business — do it! It will be one of the most gratifying feelings you will ever have. Start it with your family, but don't necessarily end it there. There are so many people who could use the help.*

A short while after the funeral, Herman's widow, Ruth, turned over the complete operation to a man I'll call Mr. B, who was the President under Herman. He was a CPA and a numbers man only interested in the bottom line. In fact, I didn't know many people inside the company that had good words to say about Mr. B, except that he was Herman's number cruncher. It didn't take long for this to become a problem for me. Every time I wanted to start a new project and talked to Mr. B and Jim about funding it, Mr. B refused. I had always gone directly to Herman on such things, and he was almost always enthusiastic about my ideas, which more often than not, turned out to be profitable endeavors. I would tell him my plan, and soon after, the funds would follow.

Apparently, this was a bit of a sore spot for Mr. B. Maybe he thought that my relationship with Herman undermined his authority. In any event, it's safe to say that he wasn't very fond of me, to say the least. Now he had his chance to get even, by stymieing all of my expansion initiatives. And when I complained about it, guess what he did? He fired me. Can you imagine? Firing the number one salesman in the company? Mr. B called me into his office and told me that he didn't want me draining the sales fund anymore with all of my ideas. I didn't understand it then, and I still don't today. Growing the business for Herman all of those years didn't drain anything, it only expanded the opportunities for everyone. Perhaps Mr. B had something else up his sleeve. Who knows? But it certainly didn't seem logical or in the best interest of the company.

I was beyond shocked. After all of my successful years with the Perl Corporation, I felt completely blindsided and wronged. So I decided to go directly to Ruth Perl, Herman's wife, and appeal to her. Although I didn't want to work for Mr. B, I had an idea. I explained to Ruth that Herman would not have agreed with what Mr. B was doing and that he would have wanted me to have the Greenwich franchise, since I had built it from nothing. I proposed that I buy all of the accounts that I had sold up until then (which were now close to 1000) for a reasonable fee, and in exchange, the Perl Organization would allow me to continue to use their monitoring station for all of my current and new accounts. Ruth acknowledged that Herman would have wanted me to own the franchise and agreed to the terms. Luckily her word trumped Mr. B's on such matters. I appreciated her fairness and was very relieved that she did the right thing by me.

King of My Own Castle

> "Strive for businesses that complement each other
> like the man who was a Veterinarian and a Taxidermist.
> Either way you get your dog back."
> — Mike Buckman

Sometimes, when you think that something is the worst thing in the world, it can actually turn out to be a gift that gets you on a completely new path. So now this was it. I was on my own, with my own business, controlling my own destiny. It wasn't necessarily by choice, but when I came to accept the situation and embrace the change, it turned out to be the single best thing that ever happened to me and my family's lives. I'll always be thankful to Herman and Ruth Perl, and of course, Mel Harris. All the years of training with them would finally pay off. Working for them with great passion and pride helped me to become a businessman and entrepreneur in my own right. That kind of knowledge cannot be found in a book. Sure, a book can give you concepts, but the practice can only be learned through experience. This would be my first time running a business without any partners. Of course, I'd made every-day decisions for all the past years in others' businesses and ran them like my own, but this was different. Now it was my turn, my money, my problems, and my total decision to build my own castle. I felt lucky to have learned how business works, how to make a profit and how to always look to the bottom line. Just talking about it gets my juices flowing.

> **Mini-Lesson:** *It always pays to pay attention and keep your head and hands on the pulse of your business.*

Life is so strange. Herman's death turned out to be a real "birth" for my family and me. If you could imagine, I worked even harder than I did before, and I pulled out all the stops to make every moment count. They closed the Norwalk office and I ran my business, with the accounts I had bought, from a small office in Greenwich. It was a walk-up on the second floor of a small shopping center, with a cheap rent that I felt I could afford. I didn't want to overextend myself right out of the gate. The office had just enough room for two desks, and not much more. We had a typewriter, a file cabinet and a phone, and when we needed to make a copy, we went next door and paid for the copies. It took us seven months to get a copy machine of our own. Around that time I added another phone line. I dutifully employed my ABCDs, and then a funny thing happened — we started to grow. The sales came fairly easy for me. Eventually I took on another salesman and added space when a room became available next door, and then I never looked back.

Sometime during 1976, my friend Barry Trupin went into the capital equipment leasing business and asked me to join him in Manhattan to meet the lawyers he was working with for lunch. Always looking for an opportunity to meet new people and make connections, I went with him and met three lawyers over a pastrami sandwich. Little did I know that they would become my friends and eventually my own attorneys later in life. Barry tried very hard to convince me to give up my alarm business and join him as a 50-50 partner in the capital equipment leasing business. I was interested and thought about it on and off over a couple of months. He was certain he was "gonna make a million dollars," and wanted me to join him as soon as possible. We were spending time with Judy and Barry almost every weekend, and I noticed that their lifestyle was visibly changing for the better. I began to think that maybe there was something there.

The alarm business was doing very well. In fact, I doubled my income in one year, but Barry continued to ask me to join him, and I was beginning to lean towards saying yes. I contacted one of my alarm clients in Greenwich, Tom Watson, and asked for his advice. Mr. Watson was a major player and the Chairman of IBM at the time. I was encouraged when he said he thought I could learn the equipment leasing business and do very well at it. Mr. Watson offered to put me on the preferred vendor list at IBM, which would be a huge help in getting our foot in the door. He introduced me to his very close friend in Greenwich, Mr. John Randolf of Randolf Computer. I went home to discuss the opportunity with my family and, God bless them, as always they were very supportive. I told them we'd possibly have to put up all our money and mortgage the house and cars plus the savings we had managed to put aside from the Levine 10% rule, and dear Fritzie was still behind me.

But there was one problem. My alarm business was too successful to give up and I didn't think it was the right time to sell. So I had a heart-to-heart with my son, Steve. Steve had received a football scholarship to Villanova University in Pennsylvania, but transferred to C.W. Post on Long Island after his first year, in order to be closer to his friends. He now had only one year left before graduation. He was also dating a girl from Long Island named Barbara Campbell, and things were getting serious between them. When I told him I had something very serious to discuss with him, he paid close attention and heard me out. It was one of the hardest things I ever had to do. I took a deep breath and calmly asked my son if he would consider quitting college and taking over the alarm business. I told him that he couldn't do it on a part-time basis — he'd have to commit to it 100%, because that's what was required to run it. I added that perhaps he could go back and finish school at a later date.

As you could imagine, this was not an easy conversation, especially because I myself always regretted not getting a formal college education, and was so proud of my son's academic and athletic achievements. Now I was asking him to give that up. Although, I truly did believe that it was the right thing to do for the company, for our family and for Steve, it was a difficult and emotional decision. Steve completely understood the situation and agreed that selling the company at that time was not the right thing to do. However, before he could decide, he wanted to talk it over with Barbara. Of course I understood, and I was even more proud of him for handling this decision with such maturity. I could see that he had really grown up, and was now a smart, thoughtful man that I was incredibly proud of and was more than ready to take on this responsibility.

I think I may have made it easier for him to say yes when I made him this offer: If he could make the company grow by 10% each year, I would give him an additional 10% ownership per year — up to 50% of the company. Talk about motivation. Steve, being as competitive and driven as his old man, was determined to make this happen. So Steve took the deal, left school to work full time and wound up loving the world of sales as much as I did. He also happened to love the business of helping save lives and property. I'm sure taking him on all of those sales calls with me when he was a kid certainly helped. I taught Steve almost everything I knew about the alarm business, and always focused on the positive elements of it.

> **Mini-Lesson:** *No one likes a rain cloud. People gravitate to the sunshine. Teach employees everything they need to know about your job. In business and in sailing, it is easier to adjust the sails than to try to direct the wind.*

So off I went into yet another career. Remember, when opportunity knocks, answer that door! There are opportunities all around you, but you have to decide to take advantage of them. Sometimes it's messy and you need to rearrange your life to accommodate them, but they are there nonetheless. Although Steve missed the 10% growth goal the first year, he worked harder than any salesman I know and swiftly increased sales by 200% and wound up owning 50% of the company even faster than anticipated. He was a natural in his first year. "Pretty fantastic!" I thought.

I, on the other hand, had to go back to school to learn about equipment leasing and the complex tax laws and restrictions that went along with it. I got a Securities Principal license, registered as a broker-dealer with the NASD (National Association of Securities Dealers) and became a member of the International Association of Financial Planners. The equipment leasing business worked like this: You bought a piece of equipment then leased it to someone else. It could be an airplane, train, ship, computer or any allowable commodity. As the owner, you were allowed to claim the depreciation, fees and interest as a tax deduction, so long as you met the criteria set by the government, and in the meantime, the lessee made the payments on the equipment. It was similar to the Net Jets model, where multiple clients pay for and make use of the same plane, which is owned and serviced by a single owner, or when a landlord uses a tenant's rent to pay off the mortgage. I believed that the reason the government allowed the deductions was to ensure that more money would be in the hands of businessmen all over the U.S., allowing them to grow and build more plants and factories and drive higher employment. Perhaps I was a little naïve, but those were the policies of the time.

> **Mini-Lesson:** *You are the person in the driver's seat and the architect of your own life and future – only you. The world changes every day, but I knew I was selling value and benefits, the only two things people ever buy. MAN, was I ENTHUSIASTIC!*

It was all very new to me, but I had good teachers. I started to learn the computer leasing business and with it, a whole new language. I now had enough confidence to believe that I could sell anything that I believed in (attitude), given half a chance and the education needed to learn about it (believability). And even though I didn't have it all pieced together yet, I trusted in my own ability to know that it would come sooner rather than later (commitment) and did the work needed to make sure that happened (discipline). Barry and I drove from Connecticut to New York and back on a daily basis, and my education started from the minute we were in the car together until we reached our destination — three hours per day of driving time and intensive learning. On top of that, I went to our attorney's office almost daily for more training on the legal aspects of the business.

We named the company Rothschild Royce, International — Barry was Rothschild, and I was Royce, as in Rolls Royce (it was my dream to own a Rolls Royce convertible one day). During the end of that first year, I only made one big sale but I hung in there (commitment, again) until one day I met an accountant who introduced me to one of his clients — a guy who wrote music for commercials named Joey Levine (no relation). Joey was a young, very successful, terrific guy, as well as a former partner of the singer Barry Manilow. Joey and I hit it off and became good buddies.

He was my first client in the equipment leasing biz and introduced me to many more. It went very well after that, and within two months, I earned more than I ever had in an entire year — over $150,000. I hadn't yet realized the potential market for sophisticated investors looking for tax-advantaged investments, or tax shelters. The words "tax shelter" meant just that: shelter your income by off-setting depreciation and interest on a piece of equipment. Our CPAs addressed the accounting questions, our attorneys addressed the legal issues and I continued to bring in potential clients, all the while trying to listen, learn and up my game.

> **Mini-Lesson:** *To get something you never had, you have to do something you never did.*

On New Year's Eve the first year, we worked until midnight, as some people couldn't make up their minds about buying and taking advantage of the deduction. Sometimes their tax attorneys and accountants reminded them that they either had to buy from us or someone like us, or pay the money to Uncle Sam. Those who didn't buy usually came back or called after April 15th the next year, after they wrote large checks to the government. There were many different types of tax shelters and many people in the business were dispensing syndicated programs that were not acceptable to the IRS. They tried everything — books, records, movies, art, windmills, and more (I was surprised that I hadn't heard of anyone trying spaceships). I knew we were one of the best companies out there, and I was very proud that we had a legitimate product on the market. Having Tom Watson of IBM as my friend and alarm system client didn't hurt either. I wound up asking him for help and advice on several occasions, and he introduced me to many great contacts.

During the week I continued to work and learn in New York City, and I spent most all my weekends helping Steve continue to build the alarm business. I loved every minute of what I was doing and didn't mind the workload, although it was intense. The growth was happening right before my eyes at such an accelerated rate that I could hardly believe it.

> **Mini-Lesson:** *The successful businessman will promise only what he can deliver and then deliver more than he promised. When you start a journey, you have to go the distance in order to make it happen.*

Fritzie's Struggle

"I have learned that success is to be measured not so much by the position that one has reached in life as by the obstacles which he has overcome while trying to succeed."
— Booker T. Washington

Around the same time that the business began to really take off, I started to have some serious problems at home. Despite her unwavering support and encouragement, the pressure of raising the kids, the many moves, the ups and downs of the businesses all took its toll on Fritzie. The truth of the matter is that after Larry's diagnosis of mental retardation Fritzie began to drink. The devastating news, plus Larry's continued struggle to develop and live a normal life weighed heavily on her, and she would use alcohol to ease the pain. Although I would occasionally wonder if she was drinking a little too much here and there, I was so focused on growing my businesses and had gone so much of the time that I couldn't (or wouldn't) see that it had developed into a real problem. But now that the kids were pretty much out of the house and she wasn't focused on taking care of them anymore, the drinking increased to a level that I could no longer ignore. I tried to broach the subject with her many times, but she would deny that she had a problem and refuse to discuss it. I felt completely helpless and frustrated.

Then one Sunday morning in the summer of 1979 I reached my breaking point. Fritzie and I had a particularly heated argument that started in the kitchen, took us all over the house and finally out to the back yard, where it culminated in me yelling, "This has got to be it. You must stop drinking and stop now, or this marriage will not last!" With that, Fritzie turned on her heels, and stormed back into the house announcing that she didn't care and was going to pour herself another drink. The next thing I remember is hearing the loud smash of a bottle shattering into the sink. At the same time, I heard a man's voice shouting, ""Stop! Don't touch that drink! Put that drink down now!" I knew no one else was in our house, so I ran inside to see whose voice it was.

Fritzie was standing in the kitchen with a look of total shock and surprise on her face. The voice was coming from the kitchen television and belonged to Oral Roberts, the famous televangelist. He then gave out a phone number, and I watched in amazement as Fritzie put down the drink, went to the phone and dialed the number. We hugged and cried. Less than an hour later, two women affiliated with Oral Roberts' organization and Alcoholics Anonymous knocked at our front door. These wonderful women took Fritzie to a meeting right then and there, and from that day on, she never touched another drink. How is that for divine intervention?

In fact, she wound up becoming a leader in the local AA chapter — a shining star and one of the true believers in helping other people. I cannot begin to tell you the amount of people that she supported and sponsored over the years. We received so many calls on a constant basis. She attended daily 7:30 a.m. meetings, where she sat next to her friends and fellow members sharing of herself without reservation. Fritzie became a brilliant communicator, giving others inspiration and motivation to stay with the program. One day at a time, every day of her life. I know it brought her great satisfaction, and I am so very proud of her. Thanks, my love, for making life better in the Levine household and so many other households.

April 1980

> *"Beware of him who gives thee advice according to his own interests."*
> *- Talmud*

Although business was good, things between Barry and I began to quickly unravel. I didn't approve of some of the questionable deals he was doing and some of the people he was getting involved with. I also thought that he was taking advantage of our arrangement and withdrawing more cash out of the business than he was entitled to. When I made that known to him, things got extremely tense and finally reached a point where we needed to dissolve the partnership. I found an office apartment at East 54th Street, not too far from our former shared offices, but just far enough, where I set up shop. It was rather hard to walk away when we were making so much money, but what came later in life for Barry makes me eternally grateful that I got out when I did.

> **Mini-Lesson:** *Be ethical and maintain your reputation at all times. It'll make the world a nicer place for you and everyone else.*

Although I don't know all of the details, Barry did go to prison regarding some of his business dealings. Who knows, if things didn't go as they did, he could have dragged me to prison with him. God works in mysterious ways. Once we decided to split the business, I preferred to have the accountants and lawyers work out the details so that I could try to stay in a positive mental state and focus on the business of selling. And that's just what I did. 1980 was a super year and I made over $350,000. I happily watched the alarm company grow and Steve become more and more settled and successful. There was no telling how far things could go.

I Love New York

1980

My hard work was paying off and the business was really picking up steam. I decided that we needed more space so the search began. Realtors showed me lots of great places — some too large, some too small and some just in the wrong location. One lucky day, a nice realtor called to tell me she had a place that was just right — The Carnegie House at West 57th Street and Avenue of the Americas. The unit in question had belonged to the pianist and record producer, Bob James. I made the appointment and went to see what would soon become my wonderful Manhattan office penthouse for the next 15 years. I walked in and just knew that this was the place. It had everything we needed to grow the business, as well as the wow factor that showed others that we were doing well.

The duplex penthouse apartment was right around the corner from Carnegie Hall and it was my pride and joy. Something I felt I had earned by working so very hard to achieve success. The wraparound terrace had 180 degrees of amazing views – Central Park, the East River, the Hudson River and Radio City Music Hall. Plus the World Trade Center all the way downtown. It had four bedrooms and 3 1/2 baths of splendor. I converted three of the bedrooms into offices, two on the 20th floor for myself, my salesmen and assistants, another on the 19th floor off the kitchen, for my various regional salesmen often visiting from out of town to use.

The master bedroom adjacent to my office became our Manhattan pied-a-terre, and came in very handy on those evenings when I had to work so late into the night that driving back to Connecticut was untenable. I felt very blessed to have such a magnificent new place, right in the heart of Manhattan. It was an exciting time. Fritzie would often take the train in from Connecticut and stay over a few days during the week or over the weekend while I worked very hard to grow the business. She enjoyed decorating our new apartment and loved getting a taste of city life in our new digs.

Building the Team

> "The next time you are having a bad day, remember that even gray skies are just clouds passing over."
> — Teddy Roosevelt

I kept another bedroom for my houseman and driver, Willie, to use on nights when I stayed in the city. The story of how Willie came to be in my employ is worth noting. As I said, business was good, and because of all of the traveling I was doing, I felt the time had come for me to have my own limousine. It seemed crazy, but I did it anyway. After a brief discussion with Executive Limousine in Long Island, I agreed to purchase a brown stretch limousine. When it was delivered the next day, the delivery driver asked, "So who's going to drive it?" In my impulsiveness, I never even thought about who would drive the thing. I went nuts trying to find a driver fast.

During the first few months of owning the limo, I hired three different drivers before settling on wonderful Willie, the best of the best. He was always punctual, kind and well-mannered — a delightful man and an excellent driver. Willie came to live in the Carnegie House with us as well as the Connecticut house all through the 1980s and part of the 1990s. He was a tremendous help to me and became part of the family. After my cancer diagnosis, when my world turned upside-down, I decided to give the limousine to a friend at MTC Limo for free in exchange for driving me at no charge for two years. It worked out great for everyone involved, and I'm very glad that I was able to help Willie plan his future after I couldn't keep him as my driver. He deserved every bit of my effort on his behalf. It was a wonderful private chauffeur position with a medical company based in New York City.

> **Mini-Lesson:** *Treat people the way you want to be treated. It will help everyone in the end.*

When my assistant Marilyn decided to retire, I placed an ad in the newspaper and had the good fortune to hire a lovely lady named Linda Keppler. I interviewed Linda and hired her on the spot due to her credentials, enthusiasm and work ethic, which I felt we needed in order for us to reach even higher levels of success. She had a great attitude and when she made the move to the Carnegie House, she not only kept up with all of my salesmen, accountants, lawyers and clients, she became an expert at juggling my hectic schedule. I was sad when I had to say goodbye to my friend and assistant after two years of service, when she sought sunshine, adventure and a new life in California. We've stayed in touch through the years as she married, had three kids, moved from L.A. to San Francisco, then to Lake Tahoe and finally to Reno, Nevada. I was very happy when she recently flew in for a visit to help with this book. Thanks for your all of your hard work, Linda. I wish you continued success as you enjoy life to its fullest.

On the Waterfront

Life was good again. Business was booming, and I earned over $1.2 million in 1980. Incredible! Plus my family was back on track. Although my normal work hours were from 6 a.m. late into the night — often until midnight — when you love what you do, it's not work. I had (and still have) a great passion for working with people, forming relationships and communicating ways to help colleagues succeed, so I was loving every minute of it. What also helped was, at Fritzie's urging, I decided to see a psychiatrist to try to get a deeper level of understanding about myself and clear Barry from my head. I had regular, wonderfully therapeutic sessions for six months, which helped me get closure on my past and enabled me to visualize an even better future for myself and my life in general.

Fritzie and I began working on what would become our annual project for the special needs children. We wanted to help get the children what they needed to make life easier for them at the Lower Fairfield Regional Center, and that spawned The Pro Sports Challenge. It takes place on the last Saturday of June every year, and has become a full family affair with Steve, the twins and their families fully involved, as well as extended family and friends.

Major corporations sponsor teams to have fun and compete against each other in various sporting events, ultimately raising money for the LFRC. Blessings to all who have participated. We've raised millions over the years, and 100% of it has gone directly to the benefit of the children. We have been able to provide them vans that have lifts for the handicapped, a swimming pool with special ramps and wheelchairs, field trips, renovated accommodations, clothes, televisions, furniture and much more. I've said it before and I'll say it again, I think the greatest satisfaction a person can get is to help another person. I've found that many avenues open up when you try to help others, like the time when I asked Tom Seaver, the baseball legend (and also my client in the alarm business), to sign a few baseballs for sale to raise money for the children. Not only did he do it, he signed 100 balls and came himself to play with the kids for a couple of hours. Thanks, Tom — you really are quite a man. You have a huge heart.

> **Mini-Lesson:** *Always remember that the good work you do does not go unnoticed. The most significant achievements that were once thought impossible can become your greatest assets. Doing good for someone becomes who you are. Your heart and your head are in sync, and chances are, your feet are also moving in the right direction.*

During the early 1980s, Fritzie and I continued to work on our beautiful home in Trumbull, Connecticut — enlarging it, building a pool, tennis court and lovely gardens. Boy, did Fritzie love her gardens — everyone was always so amazed at her green thumb. We were driving beautiful new cars, our twin girls were off at college in New England and we had some amazing vacations, including trips to Europe. We hosted an annual July 4th party which got bigger and bigger every year. The first party was in 1967 with just our family and five guests. Through the years it grew to a guest list of over 250. We always tried to make it interesting by having unique and fun invitations and themes each year. Everyone loved the giant lobsters, averaging four to five pounds each, as well as the prime cuts of steak from the amazing Stew Leonard, who is part of our family. We all had the best time.

December 1981

> "Destiny is not a matter of chance; it is a matter of choice."
> — William Jennings Bryan

Around that time a friend and client of mine from the capital equipment leasing business, Dan Pena, asked me if I was interested in going into the oil and gas business with him. Always open to new opportunities, I did some research, agreed to join forces with Dan and we wound up doing very well together. He would find the oil companies for us to partner with, and I would raise the funds. We called the company G & J, for Goy and Jew, as an inside joke, just to be funny. Great name, don't you think? Dan later moved to Scotland where he bought a castle, where he now lives and runs his investment and motivational seminar businesses. Several years ago he wrote a book entitled Your First 100 Million. I'm honored, not only that be mentioned me in his book, but that he referred to me as "the best salesman he has ever met." Thanks, Dan. We shared some fun times, and I'm glad that you've done so well. Way to go, my friend.

Things were going so well that we began thinking of upgrading and moving from Trumbull to the nearby town of Westport. Fritzie looked at a lot of houses but none of them quite suited us. We wanted a really nice place, something very special. One day, Stuart Epstein, a partner of mine in a real estate venture, suggested we call his wife Judy who was a realtor. Judy wasn't sure we'd be interested in this "mini-mansion" as she called it. She thought it might be too big, but she asked us to come and look at it anyway. As we walked in the door of the house on Bluewater Hill, the broker whispered to Fritzie, "He won't like it." How very wrong she was — I fell in love instantly! It was crazy. It looked like something out of the Great Gatsby. Never in a million years did I ever think I would be in a position to have such a house. I leaned over to Fritzie and said in her ear, "We are going to own it." She looked at me incredulously and said, "You're kidding?" I said it again. "We own it!"

The current owners had sold off the front gardens and the lot in the backyard, along with another building lot, leaving us with two acres. "Plenty of property," I thought. It still left enough to have a view of the waterfront from the back of the house. We made an offer for $670,000 cash, and Bluewater Hill was ours. At that time, I was doing about $100 million in gross business a year. It was an incredible feeling, and it was a very special piece of property. We did a title search and found out that we were the fourth owners. The house had been built in 1906 by Arnold Schlate who started a little business by the name of The Texaco Company. I thought it was a sign that at the same time I was entering the oil and gas business, I moved into a preeminent oilman's former home. It seemed meant to be. "Beshert" (meaning God's will in Yiddish).

Arnold Schlate and his partner, Buckskin Joe Collanan, built Texaco with Arnold serving as banker. He chose to build his home in Westport, Connecticut, and constructed a massive 19,000 square feet of living space. The property was originally comprised of 40 acres, including a private beach, two clay tennis courts, a bowling alley and all the conveniences possible in 1906, including an Otis elevator and a handball court on the fourth floor. German and Norwegian craftsmen built the house, and the details were incredible. In 1940, Schlate moved to Florida and sold the house to a Mr. Black, chairman of Chock Full O' Nuts. Black lived there with his lady, Paige Morton Black, until 1974, and it was said that the parties they hosted were right out of a fairy tale. For whatever reason during their ownership they sold off 35 acres of property, and the Bluewater Hill Association was formed among a group of homeowners. The Blacks eventually sold the house to a group of attorneys, and they sold it to us.

Before we moved in, we took our kids, friends and my mother to see it. Some of them thought we were crazy, some gave us encouragement and congratulations and all of them were shocked, but no reaction was better than my mom's. When I drove her up to the house, and we came around to the front entrance, she looked up and said, "Which apartment is ours?" I laughed and said, "Mom, the whole house is ours." She couldn't believe it. After a few minutes she asked if she could invite her friends. I said, "Sure!" and I saw tears come to her eyes. It was a really magical moment.

> **Mini-Lesson:** *If you have the opportunity to give back to your parents as I did, do it. The most incredible feelings came thru me. My mom's life was never the same. She always believed everything can come to those that earn it, and this was a dream realized.*

Moving Day

The house hadn't been maintained properly for several years and needed a lot of work inside and out. We didn't have the foggiest idea of what we were getting into, but we were up to the challenge. We knew we wanted a pool and patio at one end of the house down by the water, and Fritzie also thought that we needed a new kitchen. During the first year we took on those improvements as well as adding an outdoor kitchen, bathroom and changing room. There were several more pressing problems that needed our attention, however we had no idea at the time.

We were planning to have our annual Fourth of July party to show off our new home, so during that first winter of 1983-84, we spent most of our free time inside fixing things up. We really didn't go outside around the property much, but in the spring we found out that every time we flushed the toilets (in our nine bathrooms), the water would come above ground down at the waterside of the house. We learned that each time the previous owners sold off a plot of land, they had sold off the original septic system with it. When they put in a new system for the home, it was sorely inadequate. Apparently, the system they installed was barely sufficient for a three-bedroom house.

It was just about time for the big party, and the invites were sent, but we still hadn't solved our plumbing problem. The smell was terrible and the water made the ground sloshy and slippery. We needed to come up with a quick fix to make the smell and the water go away, at least until after the party. After some thought and a discussion with an architect friend, we bought fifteen 4x8 wall boards and some 2x4's to go underneath. We sprinkled 100 cases of baking soda under the boards and put strips of sod on top. Then we got the best smelling flowers, plants and bushes we could find and placed them throughout the area, and it worked! The lawn stayed dry for the duration of the party and people smelled the flowers and nothing else. No one was aware of the mess underneath. Thank God (and Joe Fuller, the architect).

> **Mini-Lesson:** *Where you are is important, but not as important as where you are going.*

Sparkling Waters

"As I go through life, I hope I can create more laughter than tears."
- Anonymous

Right after the party, we had the tank removed and hooked up the house to the town's sewer system. It was a major job that cost us $77,000. So, the great deal I thought we had gotten on the house maybe wasn't all that great after all — at least at that moment. Even though it turned out to be a bigger investment than we'd planned, I wouldn't have changed it for the world — we loved the house. My mother loved it too. She had her own wing with her own bedroom, sitting room, bathroom and large patio where she could smoke her cigarettes (unfortunately, I could never get Mom to kick the habit). We also decided to install central air conditioning, not realizing that the kitchen floor was made from 12 inches of poured concrete. It took six days for the workmen to drill the holes necessary to install the system, and the kitchen was out of service for months.

We ate out breakfast, lunch and dinner that entire first year. It was also the year we filled the swimming pool with sparkling water. Seeing the water delivery truck arrive and the amazed look that the driver gave me was priceless. He thought I was nuts, and he was right. It was definitely crazy, but what a great feeling to be able to be crazy just once. Well maybe twice. I guess I was so astounded by the amount of money I was earning at that time, that I didn't even know what to do with it. Oh well, live and learn. Luckily, as I got older I discovered much more altruistic and productive ways to spend it, but I never forgot the Levine 10% rule.

> **Mini-Lesson:** *Never stop the saving of 10% to put away for the bad time or rainy day, which of course we think and hope will never come. Keeping up is always easier than catching up.*

The Bluewater Hill house was so big that it literally required a staff to run, and our home was definitely in need of a team to help keep it running smoothly. After some business meetings in Manchester, I planned to visit Dublin, Ireland to meet an Irish couple that was referred to me by a friend for potential household staff positions. I boarded the plane and sat down next to a group of guys. They were dressed in leather, wore sunglasses and had on quite a bit of jewelry. They appeared to be members of a gang of some sort. I smiled at them and asked, "What gang are you guys in?" The man beside me laughed and replied, "We're U2!" I replied, "You're me, too? Huh?" I laughed and shook my head. When they explained that was the name of their band, I confessed that I hadn't heard of them, so we introduced ourselves and chatted the entire flight to Dublin, talking about our lives and the world we live in.

The friendliest of the group, named Bono, was kind and intelligent and warm, and when I told him upon landing that I was heading to meet a couple to hire for my home back in the states, he said, "Well, it's raining outside. You'll need a good raincoat." We got off the plane, and he took me into town to a men's store and told the clerk I needed a raincoat. "Take good care of him, he's a good guy," he said to the clerk as he left. Could you imagine!?! I did wind up meeting and hiring the wonderful

Peter and Phyllis, who soon joined our family back in Connecticut and did a great job for us.

When I returned home I casually mentioned to my daughters that I traveled and chatted with a music group called U2 and Bono, in particular. They screamed and ran around the room yelling, "Bono! Bono! You met Bono? Oh my God! Did you get a picture, an autograph?" I was sorry I didn't recognize him when we met, but since then I've come to realize what a great humanitarian and important activist he is. Our plane chat showed me a man who didn't care about the money. He cared about following his passion — music — and helping those less fortunate all over the world.

<u>Family Memories</u>

Business continued to get better, and I was spending two weeks out of every month traveling to my offices around the country. I would go from Chicago to Los Angeles to Washington, D.C. to Florida and back. I built ten offices in the US including my own. It was almost hard to believe, but that was the vision I had and I knew that I would do it one day. I loved the business, and I kept my accountants and lawyers busy. They became my friends and advisors. In February, we had a big blowout party for Valentine's Day. It was a black tie gala and a magical event with a seven-piece band in the front hall, great dancers, and lots of fun, fun, fun. Fritzie and I went overboard to make the party as perfect as possible. People came in limousines and were dressed to the nines in gowns and tuxedos.

We called the party "Valentine's Day Massacre Gasser." Then in July, we had our annual Fourth of July bash at our home, with tennis, swimming, horseshoes, exercise classes, a band, lobsters and most importantly, friends and family. We enjoyed giving tours of the house and property to friends who hadn't seen the place before. Thanks to Stew Leonard and his family for being part of our lives and making all the food arrangements.

> **Mini-Lesson:** *Growing a business is never done by one person alone. The object is to create relationships and share the good times. Heaven knows, there are enough problems that happen during the course of the year that can tear you apart. When you can celebrate, do it with gusto and gratitude!*

Our son, Steve, married his long-time sweetheart, Barbara Campell, a few years earlier on Long Island. We helped to arrange a stunning wedding for them, and it was a fantastic event. The wonderful Mel Harris even flew in, right onto the back lawn of the banquet hall — in a helicopter! The twins, who were now finished with college, enjoyed the house at Bluewater Hill just as much as we did, and we loved having them home.

Leslie had begun dating the son of a friend named Gregg Oxfeld, and before we knew it, another wedding was in the works. We belonged to Rolling Hills Country Club on the recommendation of our friends and business associates, Herb and Helen Gordon (to which we are ever grateful for bringing back TBL-12 food supplement from Australia for me — more on that later) and in March of 1983, Leslie and Gregg were married at the club in Western Connecticut. We hosted a wonderful reception for 300 family and close friends. This bash took on a life of its own — Fritzie and I went all out. It's a special experience to watch your children take their vows and begin a new life with that special someone.

By this time, Steve was engrossed in the alarm business, and it was really working for him. We had almost 100 employees, and the operation was running like a well-oiled machine. Our new son-in-law, Gregg was a graduate of the Culinary Institute of America and although he loved being a chef, the demanding restaurant business and its many hours away from home began to hurt the marriage. After careful consideration, Steve and I decided to make Gregg an offer to work at the alarm company. Gregg wasn't sure about it at first, but after giving it some thought, he decided to come on board, and eventually he became one of the top salesmen in the entire U.S. for national accounts. Kudos, Gregg!

Pomp and Circumstance

January 1984 - Washington, D.C.

Our blessings were plentiful. I had offices around the country, a car and driver and amazing colleagues and staff. Business was successful beyond my wildest dreams and I didn't think it could get any better. But it did. Thanks to my cousins Muriel and Hesh Breger, who worked at the Government Printing Office and then became the manager of Amtax Washington DC (I loved Hesh) and one of my closest friends and Washington DC attorney, Stuart Gordon, Esquire. Both were very connected to the political scene, and through them, Fritzie and I were invited to President Ronald Reagan's Second Inauguration. We were thrilled.

> **Mini-Lesson:** *Opportunity knocked again and luckily the door was wide open. If you ever have an opportunity to go to an event like the Presidential Inauguration, do it. You will learn more in one day than you might in a lifetime about selling and raising money for charity.*

We were told that we could invite another couple to join us, so I invited my friend and attorney Jerry Eisenberg and his wife, Fran. For Fritzie and I to be at the Presidential Ball and the Vice Presidential Party was far more over-the-top than we could have ever imagined. We were like two kids let loose in a candy store. We had photos taken in our formal wear to make sure to document this occasion so that we could always look back and relive one of the most incredible experiences we've ever had.

I believed in our President, Ronald Reagan, and thought he was a great man. Although I wasn't a Republican or Democrat (I had always believed in the person, not the label) I liked the job he was doing in office and thought he'd been a pretty good Governor, and a great actor before that. Sometimes I thought he was still acting, but he had a likeable manner and I trusted him. Mother Bush and brother, Prescott Bush, were clients of my alarm business in Greenwich. The gala was one for the books in every way. I thought about all the fundraisers we had done for which we raised lots of money, but this was the best of the best. None of our fundraisers could touch this extraordinary event and the dollars everyone spent buying up the memories of the Reagan Inauguration was unbelievably great.

Gimme Shelter

1986

As the new year began, we joined the world in mourning the tragic explosion of the Challenger shuttle while we counted our blessings. Although the business climate was certainly changing, Fritzie and I still felt extremely fortunate. We got to travel to Europe as well as other exotic parts of the world, including Singapore, Thailand, Brazil, Hawaii, Hong Kong, Argentina and the stunningly beautiful Iguazu Falls in Brazil. Our travel companions, my cousin Ira Fine and his wife Barbara, introduced us to the fine art of cruising and the benefits of visiting multiple locations while only having to unpack once. We took many wonderful trips together and had so much fun seeing the world with them. To top it off, Steve and his wife Barbara, gave birth to our first grandchild, the beautiful Brittney Hope, named after my father (H, for Harry). Fritzie and I were now Gram and Pop. We were ecstatic!

> **Mini-Lesson:** *All that I learned about my grandparents while living with them when I was young had no relevance until I became a grandparent myself. The feeling is like no other. You learn daily to expect the unexpected. The love of a grandparent grows daily.*

Everyone seemed happy. Businesses were doing well, people were earning more, the unemployment rate was low, mergers and acquisitions were booming and the go-go eighties were in full swing. We kept moving forward in our capital equipment leasing business and never seriously considered that the tax laws might change. But they did. It was like being in a crap game and believing that the number seven would never come up or "crap out." Not very realistic, I know, but I guess we wanted so badly for the good times to continue, that we refused to believe the alternative could happen. The 1986 Tax Act was going to put all tax-advantaged investments and tax shelters like ours out of business. The tax advantages were now only going to be available for corporations, and those too would eventually be phased out. I had no choice but to wait for the next opportunity to come along. There is nothing like working with the right folks on the right project. It's like magic.

1987 - New York City

> "We act as though comfort and luxury were the chief requirements of life, when all that we need to be really happy is something to be enthusiastic about."
> — Charles Kingsley

My son, Steve, was still running the alarm business with the family working with him and doing a terrific job, while much of my time was spent looking for another project. I tried to keep an open mind and wound up getting involved in a couple of business ventures over the next few years including (but not limited to):

- Gas Storage and Delivery
- Managing wrestlers
- Television and Film — including developing a children's game show called "Masters of the Maze"
- High Speed Video and Video Conferencing
- Air Purification Systems
- Shopping Centers
- Recording Studios
- Hydrogen Auto Supplies
- Pill Station Monitoring Service, etc., etc…

Certainly a long way from cutting and styling hair. Although some have been more successful than others, I believe that one of the most necessary ingredients for success is the ability to recognize change; time has a way of providing you with the appropriate thought or solution if you are open to it. It is called "choice." Most importantly, you need a positive attitude and the belief that it is up to you — that you can and will handle the problem and find a solution. It's the belief in yourself that will give you the confidence to move forward and make the necessary change. If you try to hold on too long, life will pass you by. Recognize the signs and take advantage of new opportunities. It's what separates the men from the boys (or girls), or the successful from the just average, they say.

Life Lesson #9 - It's Not Magic, Just Work Harder Than Everyone Else if You Want to Succeed:

Here again is where choices come into play. You have options. For instance you can chose to let yourself go out of business because of a change in the law or changes in the marketplace, or you can accept the responsibility of finding a new business that will get you excited and give you a new start (preferably with a residual income). Recognizing that change is coming and being able to adapt to it is a key to survival. Starting over is sometimes a great thing. Be ready for it, and in fact, look forward to it. Build a team of winners and invest your time and energy wisely into your various families (original, work, friends). You've got to give everything you have to give if you want the same in return.

CHAPTER TEN
The Fight

LIFE LESSON #10...

*YOU CAN'T WIN IF YOU DON'T
PLAY*

"You must do the thing you think you cannot do."
— Eleanor Roosevelt

January 1991 - New York City

As George H.W. Bush was finishing up his final year as President and the world was entering the electronic age, I began to think that something was wrong with my health. As mentioned, I'd fallen on the tennis court one day, hurt my back and soon after found myself receiving those words from Dr. Ron MacKenzie's associate. Words that sounded like a death sentence: cancer, multiple myeloma, incurable. Wow. I called several of my business partners and friends, including Marty Erlichman (Barbra Streisand's manager) and Richard Kline (of Win, Lose or Draw and Tic Tac Dough fame) and told them to go ahead on projects without me, including the TV show we were developing. But they said they would wait for me. If I died, they'd proceed, but for now, they were waiting for me to get well. That's what great friends do, and that's when I knew I had wonderful friends. They really wanted me to live and would wait for me to finish the projects we had started together, including a show called "Masters of the Maze."

I was in the hospital for 54 days the first time. I had a private nurse and my own view of the city in a corner suite in New York Hospital, which kept my dream alive — the dream that I would get well. I was constantly getting chemotherapy — 27 heavy doses of various types — and got lots of residual infections. I was back and forth to the hospital all the time after my initial 54-day stay. I went to the hospital for four days, every two weeks for an entire year. It was a horror. Over the course of that year, I had no choice but to let everyone in my offices go. I felt terrible, but there was no way I could keep the businesses going in my weakened state. I thanked them all for their service and support, gave them generous severance and retirement packages and wished them well. I only kept on my bookkeeper Amy to pay my bills and handle tax issues, as I fully concentrated on getting well, which took every last ounce of my time and energy.

I had no hair left, and vanity kicked in, so I went searching for a hairpiece. I had one made in a salon on 57th Street near my old apartment. It was great and looked like my own hair, or at least that's what I thought. Trying to keep my sense of humor, I decided to name my hairpiece "Tony" and I took "him" everywhere I went. My friend Stu Gordon and his wife Valerie from Washington came up to Connecticut to take me out to dinner one night. Stu is the same guy who flew in to hold my hand when they told me I had cancer and walked with me while they transferred me on a gurney from the Hospital of Special Surgery to New York Hospital.

Sensational Stuart is completely bald and I guess he felt the idea of "Tony" was quite ridiculous, so he asked me to leave "Tony" home so I could go out on the town as his twin brother. I agreed, although I felt naked without my "Tony". That is, until we got to the restaurant and the maitre'd asked if we were brothers. I said "Yes, we're brothers but from different mothers." From then on, I started to leave the house without my hairpiece.

That's How I Roll

Throughout my year of chemotherapy, many things happened — some good, some bad, some funny, and some just plain crazy. One day, after that particularly disheartening doctor appointment, where the doctor (who shall remain nameless) told me to get my affairs in order, I made an impulsive decision that made some people question my sanity (of course, this wasn't the first time, nor would it be the last). The treatments didn't seem to be working and my life was hanging in the balance. I decided that I had to own a Rolls Royce before I died, and I believed that I only had a few days left to do it. I had always wanted a Rolls Royce, and although I knew I would fight to the death to beat cancer, if I didn't survive, at least I would die owning my dream car. I even told Fritzie that if I didn't make it, she could bury me in it. Willie drove me from the doctor's office directly up the street to the Carriage House Motors dealership in New York City (it has since moved to Greenwich, CT). With two canes helping me along, I slowly walked into the showroom and looked around.

I was immediately drawn to a beautiful "Magnolia White" 1989 Rolls Royce Corniche Convertible with red leather interior. "I want that one," I told the salesman, pointing at the Corniche. He said, "Of course, Mr. Levine. It could be ready for you in three days." I quickly replied, "I may not have three days. I want it now." In fact, I did look like I was a man close to death. Weighing approximately 140lbs, with no hair and barely able to walk, they knew I was very serious. I offered to have the funds wired instantly, and convinced the wonderful owner, Michael Shudroff, to expedite the paperwork. An hour or so later, he and his team, Zane, Ellen and Phillip got the car ready, handed me the keys, and I was ready to drive it home to Westport.

Before leaving the dealership, a concerned Willie made me promise to drive slowly and stay right behind him. I happily obliged, and kept a close distance behind Willie and the limo. I enjoyed every minute of the ride home, and for the first time in a while, I felt optimistic about my future and the battle ahead of me. The purchase saved my soul and gave me a much needed shot in the arm. All these years later, Michael and family are still my friends, I've still got the Rolls, and I still love to take it out and drive it every once in a while.

> **Mini-Lesson:** *Sometimes you have to indulge yourself to keep the dream of life alive. I realize that not every one can buy themselves a Rolls Royce, but I bet there is at least one thing that you always wanted to buy or do that is within reach. Life is what you make it, so make it the best you can. Do something to make yourself happy and smile.*

At this point, there were more grandbabies on the scene, and my daughter Leslie and her family moved in with us. She, her husband Gregg and their kids, Sara and Andrew helped to keep me smiling during that tough time. When I would hear the pitter-patter of their little feet coming down the hallway each evening to bring me my medicine, as well as tons of hugs and love, I couldn't wait to see their little joyful faces. It still makes me smile when I remember. Sara was a magical four years old, and Andrew was in the "terrible two's." It was lively and exciting to have them there with us every day. And luckily, when I needed some peace and quiet, the house was large enough to accommodate that.

One afternoon in Westport, another chance encounter opened up a new chapter in my life. Fritzie and I attended the 1st birthday party of my colleague Howard's son. It was a warm day and I was happily observing the festivities from a chair in the backyard. That is, until Howard's grandfather sat down next to me and said, "So, who's older, you or me?" I asked his age, and he proudly said, "I'm 85 years old." I replied, "Well, I guess I'm not there yet. I'm 53." His reply was, "Wow, you look a lot older than that!" To that I responded, "Well, I feel a lot older than 53." It had been a tough year for me, recovering from cancer and all the treatments involved. I think everyone at the party that day thought I was preparing to die. I'm sure that the effects of the last year were quite evident to everyone there. Even though it was basically a "not so nice" comment from an old man, I'll never forget that day, and I vowed to never allow myself to be in that situation again.

January 27, 1992 - Little Rock, Arkansas

Two weeks after its most famous resident took the oath of office as President of the United States, we departed on our first trip to Little Rock, Arkansas. The Arkansas Cancer Research Center was the place that was the highest-rated for multiple myeloma treatment, and I was ready and willing to be healed. Of course, I had some fear of the unknown, but I arrived with the will to live and the passion to fight. I knew the ABCDs of Life (Attitude, Believability, Commitment and Discipline) worked in business, and I had shared them with so many people. Now I would have to test this philosophy in ways I had never even imagined.

I met Dr. Sundar Jagganath (Dr. J) upon arrival. He was the right arm of Dr. Barlogie (Dr. B), who ran the center. Both were amazing doctors and extremely well respected. I was asked to sign a form acknowledging that the drug they planned to give me might kill me. I smiled and signed, willingly accepting the risk, as I felt I had no other choice. The doctors and hospital took exceptional care of me. They even called the local Reformed Temple and told them of my arrival and treatments. The members of the temple were also great, and wound up bringing meals to my room and holding my hand during procedures when my family couldn't be there. Fritzie and I checked into the Guest House Inn, just off the medical grounds, and met the managers, Tom and Judy Adam, who are two of the kindest people you'd ever want to meet. They, and their staff, welcomed us warmly and helped to make our stay as comfortable as possible. To this day, I consider them all part of my family. They are more like family than you would believe. Great people. Thank you all.

We filled the days with hospital visits in the morning, then shopping, sightseeing or going to the movies. We thought it was important to continue getting out and going places — any place, really. As I got stronger we were able to do more and more in each day. Some days, I would drop Fritzie off at the mall that had her favorite local department store, Dillard's. Then I'd go over to Bauman's Men's Store, where Wayne, the owner, Rick, Shawn and all of the terrific folks that worked there would help me pick out shirts, underwear, pants and jackets. They are a great bunch of people, who showed impressive respect and caring for their customers. As I got better, I shopped more, but sometimes I would just go there to hang out with the gang, have some laughs and pass the time. I also went out and bought funny videos to watch, like Laurel and Hardy, the Marx Brothers, Abbott and Costello and more. I found that the humor helped my attitude, and my attitude gave me the will to live and look to the future.

After months of being in and out of the hospital in Little Rock the doctors decided that I would need a stem cell transplant. It was one of the first in the country. I remember asking for a phone in the hospital room, telling them I had to make a call to Monte Carlo. I visualized myself there in Monaco, playing at the craps tables and then renting a car and driving down to St. Tropez. Thinking positive is a must — you have to want life more than anything! Beating cancer is your fight. The right doctor, hospital and medicine, along with the right attitude, are all part of the equation. Turns out Monaco and St. Tropez were exactly where Fritzie and I went soon after the operation was over, and we kept driving all the way to Rome!

> **Mini-Lesson:** *Think young, strong, and alive! Act successful if you want to be successful.*

Back From the Dead

April 1992 - Westport, Connecticut

On our first trip back home from Little Rock in April, we walked into our house and the whole family was standing in the Grand Foyer waiting for us. I sat down in the chair they had for me, and they began singing and dancing to songs from The Sound of Music in front of a curtain hung to resemble a stage. It took my breath away. I felt like I'd been to war, and this was my parade down 5th Avenue. I noticed Lori was missing and asked where she was. They stepped to the both sides of the curtain, pulled it back, and there sat Lori in a rocking chair holding her new precious baby girl, Julie, born the day Fritzie and I left for Little Rock, fourteen weeks earlier! There was not a dry eye in the house, including all of the house staff and Willie, my driver.

I proceeded to feel better day by day, and my local doctor, Dr. Richard Zelkowitz (Dr. Z), agreed to work with Dr. Barlogie's program in Little Rock. Dr. Jaganaath set up everything. Dr. Z is one of the kindest men in the world. He's an extremely caring and thorough doctor that truly believes in anything that works. I had to go to see Dr. Z every week for both an Aridia Drip and a blood count checkup, which was then sent to Dr. Barlogie's team for my medical history records. Every other week and then month, I went back to Little Rock, and despite Dr. Z's hesitance to develop friendships with his patients (because the friendships would often be cut too short) we did indeed become very good friends, and had a lot of respect and love for each other. Since I hadn't planned on dying in the first place, I always considered his initial reaction to be out in left field. We still laugh together today.

This regimen went on for over a year, and my blood counts got better and better all the time. Going to Little Rock became as routine as going to Manhattan for dinner for Fritzie and me. At least that's what it began to feel like. Judy and Tom always kept our suite at the Guest House Inn ready and waiting. When they knew we were coming, they would often hang one of my personal sayings on the hotel's front signage. I never knew which one they would feature: "If You Think You Can, You Can," "To Be Enthusiastic, You Gotta Act Enthusiastic," "How Can I Help You?" and others. They made every trip to Little Rock special. They are wonderful people and we have much love for them.

On my trips to Little Rock, I would buy everything I could at the hospital gift shop and brought candy for all of the doctors, staff and patients. I was so happy to still be alive that I would basically bestow gifts on anyone and everyone who crossed my path. They called me the "Candy Man" when I came into town. My days there were consumed with hospital procedures and tests, some of which were very tough on my body. These included regular bone marrow biopsy tests needed to check the protein levels of the cancer, which thankfully continued to decline. Around this time other cancer patients from all over the world were beginning to contact me on a regular basis. Some wanted guidance on treatment options. Others wanted to hear my inspirational story, and still others asked for recommendations and referrals to doctors and medical institutions.

I'm not sure how they found out about me, but they did, and I was very happy to help. I found tremendous comfort in the phrase, "There is strength in numbers," and I think we all helped each other with our own particular perspectives. I sent hundreds of patients to the great Arkansas hospital where I was being treated and would set up dinners with them to talk them through the process, but most importantly, I tried to prepare them for what would literally be the fight for their lives. Believe me, you have no idea what you're facing until you're literally in the thick of it. However, you will win, if you believe.

Mini-Lesson: *Doing good things for others is not only the greatest thing you can do, it's the right thing to do.*

My Arkansas Family

One day while I was in Arkansas receiving treatment, my friend David Fishof called and told me to expect a call from a man named John Phillips from Rogers, Arkansas. David wanted us to get to know each other, as John had done some work for the Arkansas Cancer Research Center. We had a nice long phone chat, and I was impressed to learn that John was in the food business and had even been instrumental in helping Sam Walton bring food to Wal-Mart. John invited us to Rogers for a Razorback basketball game when I was well enough. He had his own stadium box, and it was a lot of fun.

While there, he introduced us to Dr. James Suen and his wife, Karen. Dr. Suen is one of the top otolaryngologists (doctor who specializes in head and neck disorders) in the world. It was an important day in the life of the Levines, as the Suens became our dearest family friends and an important part of our time spent in Arkansas. Dr. Suen has treated the likes of President Bill Clinton, Steven Spielberg and other celebrities, but even when he is treating your "Average Joe" patient, he makes them feel like they are the most important patient on Earth. The son of Chinese immigrants, he didn't think he was smart enough to be a doctor when he was a kid. Boy was he wrong. We've had the Suens out to visit our home in Connecticut, and we've taken vacations together through the years. We shared the same values regarding people and family, and the respect between us is something I cherish. As for the lovely Karen Suen (a true Arkansas gal), she could not be more wonderful or dear to my heart. Her and James are like sister and brother to me.

Dr. Suen asked me to give a keynote speech during University of Arkansas for Medical Sciences (UAMS) Grand Rounds at the Arkansas Cancer Research Center, and share my story of survival. This was a great honor to me. Doctors, nurses, patients, attendants, secretaries and anyone who wanted to attend contributed to the standing-room-only crowd in the auditorium. Another cancer survivor, a lovely young lady by the name of Katie Signaigo, spoke as well. The name of my lecture was "Life Worth Living" and meant every word. Man, it was an amazing experience to talk about my fight for life to so many people. So many people reached out to me, simply because I was still alive and told my story. They were all seeking the same thing — hope!

I continued to send many people to the Arkansas facility because I was so impressed with their treatment and thankful for their excellent care. However, because their top specialties were multiple myeloma and head and neck cancer, headed by the brilliant Dr. Suen, Dr. Barlogie, and Dr. Jagannath respectively, I eventually realized that people with other cancers were not necessarily best served there. I really wanted to help each cancer patient get the best treatment for their individual ailment.

Dr. James Suen saw how hard I was trying to help other cancer patients and thought he should introduce me to one of the smartest men in the world regarding medical knowledge. He was a rabbi. Imagine, a rabbi knowing all there is to know about medicine! I was surprised to hear that, but very intrigued. So I called the rabbi and he suggested that we meet. When we did, we immediately clicked and a strong friendship was born. He gave me his phone number and told me to call whenever I needed to answer a new patient's question. Apparently, the rabbi and his team conduct and find daily medical research (except for the Sabbath) and he knows every top physician in every field all over the world. He works with a very special group of people each day. They are able to identify "who wrote the book" on each disease or type of cancer as well as updated information on trials and grants. Now that's commitment!

Doctors also call the rabbi for input on certain patients they are treating. He is the most unbelievable man, working day and night to help others. I have always believed that I walk with God, but to be able to connect people in need and change their destiny like he does, is like holding a lightning rod in one's hand. This introduction has probably been one of the most important in my life, and there are literally many hundreds of patients for whom I've contacted the rabbi and shared his expertise with. They are alive, even though they aren't supposed to be, and filled with immense gratitude. I'm so blessed to be able to help change the quality of life for these patients as well as their families and friends. God has been very good to me, and I hope to continue to work with the rabbi every day of my life, as long as I can. I feel very lucky and blessed to do so. This is how I found my new unsalaried occupation. There may not be a salary, but the spiritual payback has been enormous. Thank you, Rabbi, for the opportunity to work with you.

> **Mini-Lesson:** *Don't be afraid to go out on a limb—that's where the fruit is.*

Cucumber of the Sea

Our family tried to go on with our lives as best we could. We still had parties at our home, including our annual 4th of July bash and regular family gatherings, including pizza night every Friday with all of the kids and grandkids — which totals seven — Brittney, Sara, Brian, Jamie, Andrew, Julie, and Nikki. Larry would visit from the Norwalk Center every Sunday and the kids would come by to spend time with him. They would also fly to Little Rock to visit when Fritzie and I were there for extended periods of time. I'm very proud of the way our family stood up and made things work while raising their own families. Then one fine day, Dr. Barlogie informed us that I now only needed to return to Arkansas twice a year for testing. The tears of joy were copious, from all around. I was torn between sheer joy and the fear of being away from Little Rock, as it had become such a big part of my life, but I had complete confidence in Dr. Z back home, and knew that he would continue to watch over me and keep Dr. B and Dr. Jagannath up to date on any changes in my health.

Just after my stem cell transplant, when I came back from Little Rock, my friend and former business associate in the recording studio business, Herb Gordon and his wife Helen, came to visit me in Westport. He brought me 2 boxes of these small containers, and in them was something called "TBL-12/Sea cucumber." I'd never heard of it. Herb then told me the story about how he was visiting his daughter, who was living in Australia as an exchange student, when he met a man named Sam Grant who owned a company in the Pan Region. Sam told Herb a story about what happened when he first learned that his dad was diagnosed with cancer. He was sitting on the Great Barrier Reef Beach crying when a Chinese sea captain came up to him and asked, "Why are you crying?" Sam answered, "I was just told that my dad has stomach cancer and doesn't have long to live." The sea captain replied, "He doesn't have to die." Sam asked, "How would you know, you're just a sea captain."

The Chinese man said, "I have a problem with my boat's engine. If you can help me fix it, I'll mix something up for your dad and make a batch to last six months." Well, Sam's family was in the boat repair business, so he told him he'd fix it. He came to find out that sea cucumber is an animal, not a vegetable, and the sea captain told him that people from his country had been coming to Australia for centuries to harvest them, plus sea urchins, sea squirts and marine grasses to use as dietary supplements. "Take it with you. It will help your father," he said. Sam's dad starting taking it in 1972 at age 52 and he wound up living well into his ninety-first year. Herb told me that he started taking it too. "Nothing bad happened to me, and it actually helped my arthritis. I definitely feel better," he added. Herb said that the first two boxes was his gift to me and he hoped that it would help. They made me promise I would take two every day. After it was finished, I was free to buy more. I did, and I still take it every day. I never miss a day whether I'm home or travelling. I attribute my great health to the TBL-12/Sea Cucumber, and I will never stop taking it.

When the doctors got my latest blood results and saw that my counts had dropped faster than any of his other patients he wanted to know why. I told him about the sea cucumber and he asked me to bring it in. When I did and he smelled it he told me that I was nuts. However, he also told me to continue taking it and the truth is, I haven't been without it for one day since I started taking it in May, 1992.

> **Mini-Lesson:** *If you find something that you believe in, whether it be religion, faith, a friend or a product (even a dietary food supplement like TBL-12/Sea Cucumber), try it. What have you got to lose? Many doctors feel the same way.*

Soon after that, the comments from friends, acquaintances and family have been much different from the sentiment that 85 year old Grandfather expressed to me that day at the birthday party. I'm told often and with great enthusiasm, sincerity and surprise that I don't look anywhere near my age and that I literally have a glow of health about me. In fact, I'm told all the time that I look no older than 60-ish, and I feel like I'm 50!

My life has changed so much since beating cancer and beginning the daily regimen of TBL-12/Sea Cucumber, which was (and still is) a huge part of my recovery. I believe that the supplement has anti-aging and anti-oxidant properties that keep my immune system strong and make me feel vibrant and alive. My body has been free of cancer for many years, and I decided that I would try to help as many others as I could to get access to the supplement, so I have operated a not-for-profit company to import and distribute the supplement to others and do my best to get the word out about it. I've been able to help people from all over the country, and I believe that it has kept many alive for many years. I love the feeling.

> **Mini-Lesson:** *Follow your heart in the direction that you believe in. Sometimes being obvious is the most effective way to get your message across, because sometimes that is what is needed to get people to feel.*

I am in the process of working with several major health institutions to have a medical trial done on TBL-12/Sea Cucumber. We are well on our way to hopefully conclusively and scientifically proving its effectiveness and have about 85% stability in the trial so far, which, from what I understand, is almost unheard of. My vision is to have it officially approved for use by the medical community so that it can be manufactured and marketed by one of the large pharmaceutical companies. Only then can it get the widespread distribution needed to provide everyone with the benefits of this miracle product, which I believe helped save my life.* The insurance companies want to keep people alive so they can pay their premiums and live forever — maybe they will co-pay for it. This is my goal.

*Disclaimer: The product TBL-12/Sea Cucumber, is a dietary supplement that has been used for many years by the people of Asia for all types of health-related issues. The product itself is not FDA approved at the time of this writing, but will hopefully be soon, as it is being tested in several medical trials, which are FDA approved. Currently, it is considered a dietary food supplement only and is NOT a prescribed medicine. At this time it is only available for purchase through this website: www.sea-cucumber.com. I cannot guarantee any results from the use of TBL-12/Sea Cucumber, but I do personally believe that it helped me and many others in our fight against cancer.

Yiddish Mamma

1993 - Westport, Connecticut

Fritzie and I recently returned home from a stint in Little Rock, and some friends convinced us to get out of town for the weekend to enjoy the "Concerts in the Berkshires." The thought of listening to beautiful music played by talented orchestras in a lovely setting sounded just perfect, so we agreed. Leslie, Gregg and the kids, who were still living with us at the time, were happy to see us take a road trip to the mountains, and they assured us they'd hold down the fort and take care of Mom while we were away. They wished us a wonderful weekend, and off we went, enjoying the novelty of such spontaneity and the promise of a little night of music in the mountains. On Friday night, Leslie and Gregg took Mom and the kids out to dinner, and had a fine time. Mom said she didn't feel like going to the ballgame they were planning to attend afterwards, so they dropped her off at the house, and they went on their way.

Meanwhile, we finally arrived in the Berkshires after a long drive, and we were trying to get some rest before attending our first concert. I remember having this strange feeling and an urgent need to call home. When I did, my daughter, Leslie, answered the phone and delivered to me the devastating news that my mom had died. The words didn't register for a moment. I was stunned and cried. Fritzie had the same reaction when I told her what had happened. We were in shock.

Mini-Lesson: *Life is hard, but also wonderful. Do not take it for granted. Make every day the very best and live life with love and gusto.*

We told Leslie that we were heading right home, and I vaguely recall knocking on our friends' door to tell them the news. We grabbed our bags and somehow drove home through our tears as we shared memories and stories of Faye on the way. My Mom was one of the greats. She was a very kind person who happily helped strangers and friends alike, and most of all, was cheerfully and selflessly devoted to her family. Faye Butler Levine was one tough lady but we always knew how much she loved us. She made it very clear that her family brought her joy and tremendous pride, plain and simple. Larry had a special place in her heart, and she cared for him more like he was her son than her grandson, letting him sleep in her bed when he spent the night, and watching television together for hours. Whatever Larry needed, my mom was there for him.

We arrived home at midnight and every light in the house was on. The kids were up waiting for us and they told us what happened. They arrived home from the baseball game, and saw Mom on the floor. She had suffered a heart attack. They called an ambulance, which came immediately, but she passed away soon after arriving at the hospital. When I became very sick with cancer, I remember Mom telling me more than once that she didn't want me to die before her. Her words kept running through my mind in the hours after her death. In the tough moments that followed her death, planning her funeral and memorial service, I kept thinking of those words and felt some comfort in the fact that she got her wish.

We put together a nice celebration of her life and had everyone back to our house afterward. We sat Shiva and received visits from family and friends to offer their sympathy and friendship. I will always be appreciative of that support and love during that tough time. Losing one's beloved mother can hurt your heart like nothing else, as those of you who have been through it know so well. My kids were sad but strong and joined in the celebration of the life of their wonderful grandmother. We shared stories and laughter and remembered the wonderful life of a kind and loving woman.

Mom and her two sisters Syd and Bea were known in the family as "See No Evil, Hear No Evil and Speak No Evil." I smile whenever I think about them. When they were together, they all looked so sweet, gentle and kind at first glance. No one realized until they opened their mouths that my sweet mother and aunts had the wildest vocabulary one could ever imagine. They were raised in a tough neighborhood in Maspeth, Queens, and then Brooklyn, New York, and like water from a fire hydrant, their gutter mouths flowed when called upon. The Butler sisters were unique. Their love of life and family was enormous.

> **Mini-Lesson:** *Keep your face to the sunshine and you cannot see a shadow; but if you do, look at the shadow with gratitude.*

But after my mom's memorial service, I continued to have a gnawing feeling in the pit of my stomach as I sat in the house reflecting on her. Her words repeated in my head, the statement she'd made, "I don't want you to die before me." I walked down the hall to her room and looked in her medicine cabinet. As I've mentioned in earlier chapters of this book, my mom had suffered several heart attacks, and the doctors were very clear with her about continuing the daily pills she needed to maintain her heart's health. I opened the cabinet and, sure enough, I found all of her prescription bottles were full. I realized then that my mom had stopped taking her pills.

My mother had lived with us for 27 years and I knew her very well. I knew at that moment that my mom had found a way, her way, to make sure that I didn't die first. Mom, if you can hear me, I'm telling you my journey is not over, not by a long shot. I'm sorry you didn't live to see more years but you had your agenda and did what you had to do. I hope your ears are ringing in Heaven because we talk about you all the time. Thanks from all of us who loved you and for all that you did for us.

There's never been a more giving mother and grandmother, and we cherish the many memories we have of you and keep you forever in our hearts. Mom, I love you. Thanks for loving me so well. There will never be another like you. As the song goes, "My Yiddish Mama, I miss you more than ever now…"

Author! Author!

"All of our dreams come true, if we have the courage to pursue them."
— Walt Disney

Relationships can start (or re-start) anywhere and at any time. You just never know, but if you don't take the first step by saying "Hello," it definitely won't happen. It gets back to treating people the way you want to be treated. One afternoon, I got on a plane to California and introduced myself to the man seated beside me. It's a six-hour flight and of course, everyone is different, so you never know if the person next to you wants to talk, read, close his or her eyes, etc. But the man next to me was happy to chat. A few minutes after we met, he asked what I did for a living. I told him, "I do everything!" My new friend, Mr. Klein, then asked, "Do you manage writers?" I replied that I had never managed a writer before, but always wanted to keep my options open and listen for opportunity knocking, I asked what he had in mind.

He proceeded to tell me about a well known, successful children's book author and illustrator in Australia named Michael Salmon, who was looking for a manager in the U.S. I laughed and said, "Here, take my card and give it to Michael." We had a wonderful flight chatting and getting to know each other further, but I didn't think much about it afterwards. That is, until one day I received a call from a man with a heavy Australian accent. Yes, it was Michael Salmon calling me from Australia. We spoke for over an hour, and I learned that at that point Michael had written and published over 100 books working with Penguin Books, and he had also lectured all over Australia. Michael told me that Mr. Klein was impressed with my enthusiasm and entrepreneurial spirit, and recommended that Michael consider hiring me as his agent here in The States.

Before long, Michael and his wife Jan came to Connecticut to visit, and we did in fact strike up an agent/writer agreement. I made some calls and spoke to a few people trying to find the best way to proceed. Then I realized, the solution may be right down the street. One of my neighbors was Marty Davis who ran Simon & Schuster at the time, so I set up some time to stop by his house (which he was in the process of completing) and meet with him to get some advice. I brought with me just a few copies of the many books Michael had already written and published in Australia. They were all very engaging stories that were richly and colorfully illustrated. Michael truly is extremely talented. Marty took a look and was so impressed that he immediately set me up with the person in charge of children's books at his company. I was able to get a contract for Michael to write eight new childrens books with a $50,000 advance (out of which I received a $5000 agent's fee), and they agreed to promote and distribute the books throughout the U.S. How exciting! I was a successful agent for a phenomenal writer. What a great start.

> **Mini-Lesson:** *It will always be in your best interest to try something new if you feel it in your heart. It takes years to become an instant success. Persistence works. You need to believe that you can do it before anyone else will.*

But, what happened next was disappointing. Before the books were published, my friend and neighbor, Marty Davis passed away and the lovely lady in charge of the children's books left the business. The company chose not to pursue it further.

As for Michael Salmon, he has now written and published a total of 161 books and is a major force in children's books throughout the Pacific Rim. Nothing ventured, nothing gained. Although it didn't work out exactly as I had planned, I don't regret taking on a new challenge and jumping into the publishing game. Perhaps on some level, it's what motivated me to put my life down on paper. Who knows?

> **Mini-Lesson:** *If you don't ask, you probably won't receive.*

<u>Downsizing</u>

1994 - Westport, Connecticut

Although Fritzie and I loved the house on Bluewater Hill, it took a lot to keep it running smoothly, and now that Leslie, Gregg and their family were in their own place, we decided it was time to sell the big house and find a smaller place to live. We put our house on the market and a buyer showed up and fell in love with it fairly quickly. He happened to be the Chairman of London Fog, and we decided to accept his offer. I thought a lot about leaving this fabulous house with its 33 rooms, the house that gave life to us for years. We treated the magnificent home with great respect, but now it was time to downsize in order to simplify our lives.

> **Mini-Lesson:** *Learn and accept when it is time to move on. It will make you stronger and open you up to a great new future. And don't forget to do it with excitement!*

Fritzie's realtor friend told her about a special piece of property available on the water on Beachside Avenue. Apparently, an older couple had just recently passed away within a few months of each other. The woman of a heart attack, the man, ironically of multiple myeloma, and the four children wanted to sell the property quickly. We went to see the property and fell in love with it instantly. It was 3 ½ acres right on the Long Island Sound with four structures on it. The main house needed a lot of work and the greenhouse was half standing, but I could see the potential. There was also a small garage and a separate cottage. They had five offers on the property at around $5 million, but each offer had a contingency. I told the realtor and the family that we could close tomorrow at noon with a cashier's check for $2.5 million in cash with no contingencies whatsoever, and they said yes. It was such a fantastic buy, I could hardly believe it. We closed the very next day, and we were the proud owners of yet another dream house on the water. This time, with its own private beach.

However, everything is not always as it seems. The house needed more work than we anticipated, and after almost $150,000 in expenses trying to fix it up, we decided that it was best to knock it down and start over. It was a big step and I still can't believe we did it. After over a year of architects, builders, furniture storage, decorators and more, we were finally ready to move into our wonderful new home. The only one we built from the ground up.

Working on this major renovation project while balancing my treatments in Little Rock demanded all of my attention and visualization skills. It was a true testament to attitude and commitment, and really forced me to put my money where my mouth was. Fritzie and I christened the house on Beachside Avenue as Gan Eden, the same name that nice lady in Greenwich had used for her home years earlier. It was our wonderful oasis, and everything I'd worked hard to achieve in my lifetime. We built a tennis court, a swimming pool and jacuzzi, a fish pond and a guest house — for guests! We even put in a putting green and a driving range. Plus I built an office in the expanded greenhouse.

Around this time, my granddaughter, Nikki, the last of the Levine family of grandkids, was born. When I got the news, I was so excited to get to the hospital and see her for the first time, that I put the car in reverse and hit a tree. I bent the back of the car and broke the window (oops). Life is great, but sometimes it can throw you a curve ball. When I got to the hospital and saw my new lovely granddaughter, I dreamed about tomorrow, and was filled with hope. Welcome sweet Nikki. Getting the car fixed was certainly worth the celebration of your arrival. Next time I'll check the rear view mirror.

People Management

I continued to keep busy with my numerous projects, when through an alarm company client, Vince and Linda McMahon, I came to know the professional wrestler, Sergeant Slaughter who was with WWF at the time. Sarge wanted to broaden his horizons and become more entrepreneurial, so he asked me to manage his career. I told him I couldn't even manage myself very well, but before I knew it, I agreed to an arrangement. While working with Sarge, I met another wrestler named Tito Santana who asked me to manage his career as well, and before I knew it, I was a full time wrestling manager. I traveled with Sarge and Tito, making deals on their behalf. I certainly met a lot of interesting people in that business, including the wrestlers Greg Valentine and Mr. Perfect, who became regular guests at our home. They were a real colorful cast of characters, who came into my life at exactly the right time. It was great fun. Let me tell you, managing wrestlers can really take your mind off of cancer — which was the idea. I wanted to keep busy and not think of the treatments and taking the TBL-12/Sea Cucumber daily as my back up.

Meeting and breaking bread with Vince and Linda McMahon of WWE (World Wrestling Entertainment) led to many more business and personal relationships — not only with their wrestlers, but with the entire organization. What an energetic group of people and brilliant promoters. I think it's just amazing how a husband and wife could build such a great franchise together. They are both ultimate entrepreneurs and experts at making shrewd decisions.

During one of my trips, I was standing in the VIP lounge at the Mirage Hotel in Las Vegas, when Mr. Steve Wynn walked in and said "Hi, Walter." We have known each other for many years. Steve, a paragon of the hospitality industry, has launched and run many successful hotels and resorts. Steve and I struck up a conversation, talking for two hours straight. I felt like we had been friends all of our lives. Steve has a special kindness that makes you feel that way. Although there are so many places to stay in Vegas, I always choose to stay at one of his hotels, as his team, including Charlie Meyerson, Steve Battaglini and Michelle Rapose definitely live by the creed of "How Can I Help You" when it comes to their clientele. Their level of service is outstanding, and they always go the extra mile to keep their guests happy. Steve is also a very generous soul who has done a lot for multiple charities, and has helped me out more than once with my various causes. In my opinion, The Wynn and Encore hotels are the best in the world. Vegas is a special place because of Steve Wynn.

> **Mini-Lesson:** *Life is built around relationships and when you use them for the benefit of charity they have a way of building excitement for what might happen next — especially when it's out of your comfort zone. Get inspired!*

On that same trip, I also had to fly to Los Angeles. I brought some peanuts from my room to eat on the plane and found myself sitting next to a very nice man, who I introduced myself to, and I offered him some nuts. We had a great conversation where he told me that he worked for a big Golf Company and had invented a very important golf club. I wasn't an avid golfer at the time, so this didn't mean much to me, but I shared with him that my wife had recently had arranged for me to have golf lessons with a local golf pro, John Cooper over at Longshore Golf Course in Westport, Connecticut, because I could no longer play tennis due to a crushed vertebrae from the cancer.

Anyway, we continued to chat. His name was Glenn Schmidt and when he asked me what I did for a living, I told him that I managed wrestlers. Out of the blue, he looked at me and asked if I would be interested in managing him. The funny thing about life is you never know when something great is going to fall in your lap, so you should always be prepared. Glenn told me he was presently upset with the owner of the Golf Company, because he believed he was never properly compensated for inventing a "Big Club," which he said became the most popular golf club in the world at the time, and was considering a lawsuit.

By the end of the flight, after listening to his story, I agreed to manage him and suggested that we put together a team of lawyers to move the case forward. I told him that I had worked with two great litigators, one in L.A. and another by the name of David Jarolsowitz in New York. I suggested we get them on board. Glenn seemed to like what he heard, and excitedly promised me 10% of whatever we got from the deal outside of his salary. We did wind up settling the case for Glenn, and he received over $40 million. Glenn paid the two lawyers I hired what he owed them, but because I trusted his word and never thought to put our arrangement in writing, I only wound up getting a $50,000 payment, plus a cool red golf cart that I used on my property practically every day. I call it my $4 million golf cart, because that was the amount of the settlement that I was truly entitled to.

I'm still very trusting of people, but I now know that in business, you do have to put everything in writing. I guess ya gotta learn sometime. Years later, I found out that Glenn moved his family to Texas, developed cancer and died soon after. I sure wish he would've come to me for help once again. Who knows if I could've saved him, but at the very least I would've been happy to offer him whatever I could, including the amazing TBL-12/Sea Cucumber, some hard-earned advice and of course, hope! The song, "People" by Barbra Streisand comes to mind.

> **Mini-Lesson:** *Knock, knock. Does that sound familiar? If you open it, a new life could begin. You can't keep doing the same thing over and over and expect different results. Do the right thing the first time and put it on paper — legally. No verbal promises, okay?*

1995

With my hard-working and smart son at the helm — and both sons-in-laws Greg and Ray on the team — the alarm company had by now grown into a national, multi-million dollar machine — with over 100 employees and about 15,000 residential and commercial clients. Nothing ever stops for long in my life, and after growing into one of the top 100 alarm companies in the country, we decided to sell. When Steve told me that we had a very good offer and we should take advantage of it, I agreed and we closed the deal. I continued to keep busy managing the wrestlers, the oil and gas partnerships and any new prospects that crossed my path.

> **Mini-Lesson:** *Remember, you can sell your business, but you always keep your name, reputation and relationships.*

One of the new prospects involved a high-speed video conferencing technology that was presented to me by Mike Maresca, a bright young television engineer. When he explained to me how it worked, I was very impressed. It was basically real-time video over phone lines enabling people to have meetings and conversations via television without having to leave their offices or homes. Back then, this was a revolutionary concept and I was sold. Mike needed help setting up the business, researching and navigating the patent process, fundraising, establishing office space, etc. and asked me for help and money. I thought it was a great idea and wrote a check to get the business started. High Speed Video (a simple and straightforward name) is a great product that works easily and well, and does it better than other systems that could cost much more.

Mike and I gathered a team of people, and I proceeded to raise the $5 million of capital for the new venture called High Speed Video (HSV). After I took the reins as Chairman, with Mike as President, we opened offices in New Jersey and Washington, DC as a connector. We started to grow quickly. Our first big account was the National Football League, and we soon went from red to black in short order. Plus we had raised enough capital to run HSV for five years. I'm happy to report that the business is still going strong to this day. We received a patent and 16 claims in various countries, and continue to add new clients regularly. As of this writing, we also handle Major League Baseball and a slew of other large corporate accounts, providing our happy clients exemplary dedication and results. We provide a valuable service to our customers by allowing them to cut down on their need for travel with real-time video conferencing. How great is that? Today we even do real time video over laptops.

Another venture that I've become involved with is the "Pill Station Monitoring Service" through the Senticare Company that started with my very good friend, Bob Russell. Bob and I have had lots of fun working together on this remarkable product created by Dr. David Bear from Harvard University and his associate, Yo Gandra. It has the possibility of saving over 340 lives a day, in the United States alone, and that is how many people die in the United States every day because they accidentally forget to take their medication, or they take the wrong dosage.

I'm so pleased to have been involved in raising the initial capital to build this product, which consists of a group of small boxes that literally tells a person to take his or her pills on time. An automated voice says, "It's 7 AM, take your pill." If the pill is not taken, it repeats the message and continues repeating it until you do. If you still don't take your pill, the service phones you (at home or even on your cell phone) with another message to take your pill, and if it still gets no response, it will phone your next of kin and finally your doctor. The concept borrows many principles from the security and alarm business, which of course, I have plenty of experience in. To me, this is an innovative, life-saving product that would be of great help to the over 100 million people (just in the United States) who need to take daily medication in order to stay alive and healthy. It can provide a huge value and benefit to many. I hope that it will soon be available to you. Thanks to Michael Staw for stepping up to the batter's box as President of Pill Station Monitoring Station, and driving its future forward.

> **Mini-Lesson:** *When you find a way to offer a product or serve that could save money, lives (or especially both), you will have the magic going on for you. Eliminate the fear of starting a business and limiting yourself from growth. Get out there and network your relationships.*

My Life's Work

> "I am a little pencil in the hand of a writing God who is sending
> a love letter to the world."
> — Mother Teresa

One day, I received a call from Mrs. Bernadette Coomaswarmy, of Greenwich, CT. Bernadette is a local judge and had been a client of my security company for many years. Her husband, Dr. Rama Coomaswarmy, was the Chief of Thoracic Surgery at Mt. Sinai Hospital in Manhattan, and had been suffering with multiple myeloma cancer. It seemed that the doctors in New York City had given Rama as much chemotherapy as they could, and they now told him to go home and get his affairs in order. Now where have I heard that before? Bernadette asked if I would talk to her husband about my survival of multiple myeloma. Of course, I agreed. Rama was a little resistant, as he was a physician and trained to be cautious, practical and scientific. I spoke in a positive manner about beating cancer, as I always do, like it was an easy feat. I don't believe that there is any good in dwelling on the hardships of the fight. It helps no one, particularly the patient. After I spoke with them they agreed to a visit with Dr. Barlogie in Little Rock to hear what he had to say.

I also suggested that Rama begin taking the TBL-12/Sea Cucumber supplement right away. They went to Arkansas, got examined and proceeded with the aggressive treatment recommended, including a stem cell transplant. They remained in Little Rock for several months, but we stayed in close touch, and visited with them both in Little Rock and in Connecticut whenever we could. In getting to know Rama better, I found out that he was from India and was Mother Teresa's first volunteer. I also learned that not only was Bernadette a judge and attorney, but in fact, she was Mother Teresa's attorney. They all laughed when I asked, "What could Mother Teresa possibly have done so wrong to need an attorney?" We all chuckled together at that idea. Then Bernadette explained that the Missionaries of Charity organization needed special clearances in order to operate legally within the U.S.

Rama and Bernadette were very gracious and grateful to me for helping them and asked if there was any way they could reciprocate. I told them I needed nothing and was just happy to help them, but after thinking about it and speaking with Fritzie, we had an idea, and decided we had nothing to lose by asking. So we asked Rama and Bernadette if Mother Teresa would consider visiting with the special children from the center where Larry lived the next time she was in the U.S., and say a prayer with and for them. The next thing I knew, Mother Teresa sent me a personal note thanking me for all of the work I was doing to help people and telling me that she would be happy to visit the center and was looking forward to meeting me. Needless to say, I was flabbergasted, honored and beyond excited! The meeting was one of the major highlights of my life.

Life Lesson #10 — You Can't Win if You Don't Play:

Faced with the biggest struggle of my life, I chose to not only fight, but to fight with everything I had. I was not going to let cancer win. I thought to myself: "Look around you. People love you. Don't give that up." Winning was the only choice. I truly believed that I controlled my own destiny (and still do). For me, my commitment to living and beating cancer was a no brainer. The mind is the most powerful tool you have. I used mine to help me live. You can too!

Part Three

CHAPTER ELEVEN
How Can I Help You?
The Most Important Question in Business and in Life

"Love is a fruit in season at all times and within reach of every hand."
- Mother Teresa

June 4, 1996 - Bronx, New York

*O*ne miraculous day, we received word that Larry, Fritzie and I, along with some of the special residents of the Lower Fairfield Regional Center, would be taken to the Bronx chapter of Mother Teresa's organization for a personal visit and prayers. The Westport News was the only newspaper I invited to take pictures and be inside the church, sitting next to Fritzie's best friend and co-hort, Cindy Stramandinoli. Cindy has worked so hard her whole life for the special kids, we were so happy to have her there to enjoy this special moment.

Into the room walked several priests and nuns, and in the middle was a tiny, 4'9" woman who stood out clearly among them. It was her, Mother Teresa. It seemed to me almost as if she had a halo over her head. I couldn't believe that I was in the presence of this world-renowned Nobel Prize winner and wonderful human being. Fritzie and I and everyone with us were completely awe-struck. We believed (and still do) that we were in the presence of a saint.

The mass began, and it was an absolutely beautiful service. After the mass, Mother Teresa continued to stand and seemed to be praying intensely. When she was finished, it was finally time for her to spend some private moments with our special children from the center near the back of the church. One child was screaming and crying. She went over to him and put both of her hands on his head. She was so calm and exuded such warmth, that he immediately stopped crying and just looked at her. She laid a hand on each and every one of the children, with a kind, loving touch and a gentle, caring look in her eyes. When she touched our son, Larry, it was almost as if he knew that this tiny 86 year-old woman reaching out to touch his hand, was family. It was such a spiritual, holy and purely magical moment, full of strong emotion.

Being raised a Jew on the streets of Brooklyn did not prevent me from being humbled in her presence. I simply could not take my eyes off of this little Catholic nun, who seemed to me the closest thing to a saint on earth. What happened next was one of the most powerful experiences of my life. When I held Mother Teresa's hand, I had a feeling like nothing I'd ever felt before. I looked into her eyes and I felt as if she was looking into my soul, infusing something in me that I'd carry with me forever. I'd had the will and desire to help others, but after receiving the personal note from Mother Teresa and now meeting her in person, I had a renewed outlook and passion.

I thought to myself, "If she can do it, I can do it." It reinforced my mission and made me want to try even harder. Everything that she represented to the world came to life inside me at that moment. She blessed me as well as the medal with her image that I wear around my neck and never remove. All in attendance were overwhelmed by the love and prayers Mother Teresa shared with us that day, and we all felt blessed to participate in this once-in-a-lifetime opportunity.

The next day when the story and pictures were published on the front page of the Westport News, our phone didn't stop ringing. Everyone wanted to know the details about our meeting with Mother Teresa. It would have been easier if we'd rented out an auditorium to tell the story once, but I must admit that I enjoyed reliving it over and over with every telling. One of the many calls I received was from Kenneth S. Lewis and Joanna Laufer, two writers who were penning a book called Inspired: The Breath of God. They wanted to talk to me about my experience with Mother Teresa for possible inclusion in their book. I was gratified to be asked and honored to contribute to their book. They did include me in their book and it was great to be asked to speak about it at Barnes & Noble to a very large audience.

I thought of how proud of me my parents would have been. It was a blessed experience that proved to me again that anyone can make great things happen in their life. All you need is the passion and desire to be a person who makes a difference in others' lives. It comes back to the all important question: *How Can I Help You?* Of course, your attitude, believability, commitment and discipline all contribute to making that happen. Mother Teresa said, "Do not wait for leaders; do it alone, person to person." I thoroughly agree. The opportunities are everywhere. Most of the time, you just have to open your eyes and do it.

Thank you so very much, lovely Bernadette, for arranging this very special experience, and dear Rama, thank you for believing in me and for taking your daily dose of TBL-12 that you said, "really made the difference in your life." I'm sorry that your kind and generous heart gave out after twelve years of fighting back against your cancer. Thank you both for your wonderful friendship. A saint came to the Bronx one day and blessed God's special children, and we were privileged to have been a part of it. I think everyone in the church with us felt the same life-altering feeling, and the belief that somehow we'd just seen the face of God. Approximately one year after that day, Mother Teresa left this world to join the ranks of the angels. I'm eternally grateful for the experience and the inspiration she provided. The framed news article, personal letter and photos of our meeting are hung proudly in my office, and remain a constant reminder of that special visit and the close bond of love and friendship between Bernadette and I, which shall remain forever.

The Man Next Door

2000 - Westport, Connecticut

I lived under the radar all my life, and then one day the radar moved in next door. When Don Imus, the controversial radio and cable television personality and author, moved next door to our Westport home, I had no idea how very much my life would be affected. I'd never been a listener or viewer of his shows, so I didn't know much about him when we met in the backyard. He and his lovely wife, Deirdre, and son Wyatt would occasionally enjoy playing on our putting green and driving range. One day, my son Larry lost the key to our golf cart and Don amused everyone by getting down on his knees and scouring the lawn to help look for it. Don said, "I can find anything in the grass." We all laughed, but we never did find the key. Don helped push the golf cart all the way to the garage, cracking jokes the whole way and demonstrating his strength and kindness. He was always very kind, as was Deidre and Wyatt to Larry. In fact, they went out of their way to help Larry when they could.

The first dinner we all had together was a learning experience. You see, Imus and his family are vegetarians and very particular about what they eat. We knew that, and Fritzie worked very hard to find an array of vegetarian delicacies that she was sure they'd like. She shopped for several days at vegetarian specialty stores and prepared a fabulous, meatless feast. However, minutes before dinner was about to be served, Imus's staff from next door arrived in their golf cart with an entire meal already prepared. I guess they didn't want to take any chances. We had so much food that we asked if it was okay to invite my son, Steve and his family to eat with us. They said "fine," and we all had a good time. In fact, Don was so comfortable in my house that he fell asleep on our couch while holding his son. It was a very sweet ending to what turned out to be a great evening. If I didn't think I'd get in trouble the next day on the air, I would have taken a picture.

Then again, I found myself often getting into "trouble" with Imus. He'd regularly tell playful tales about me on the air, going off on some tirade or another about his "crazy" neighbor Walter Levine. I started to become a listener of his WFAN radio show as well as a viewer of his MSNBC television simulcast. Friends would call me up, sometimes at the crack of dawn, to excitedly tell me that Imus was talking about me on the air again. Whenever he mentioned me and the help I was providing to cancer patients I would get inundated with calls from people all over the country asking which doctor to consult for their particular disease, and when Imus spoke about the TBL-12 sea cucumber supplement that he took for a while and expressed that he felt fit and had tremendous energy from it, cases were being ordered with great results (even though he did call it "fish guts" on the air).

He even mentioned me when he was on the Larry King Show one night. He told Larry an amusing story of the elephant statue his son noticed in our front yard. On one of our trips to Thailand, I got to ride an elephant and loved it. Ever since, I wanted to have them around me all the time. When I got sick, I received many elephant gifts from well wishers. If the trunk was up, it was a sign of good luck. If I received an elephant with the trunk down, I thanked the person but returned it to them. I felt that I needed all the good luck I could get and avoided taking a chance on any downward facing trunks. The calls from my friends and family watching The Larry King Show started almost immediately. My phone was ringing off the hook. "Are you watching Larry King? Don Imus is talking about you." It just so happened that I was watching and listening, and I was very surprised to hear my name mentioned. I smiled knowing that Larry King is also a guy from Brooklyn, just like me. Imus even suggested to Larry King on the air that he have me on as a guest.

At one point Imus needed a doctor, so he called me and I called the Rabbi to get the right referral. The Rabbi recommended a specialist in New Haven, CT, which I passed on to Don. He was very happy with the treatment and even mentioned it on his show. I also gave Don Dr. Ron McKenzie's contact information in case he wanted to use him as his personal physician. From that moment on, I was inundated with calls and emails from people contacting me to ask for my help and advice. I was very happy to be able to expand my reach and help as many people as possible. It felt great. I thank you Rabbi for being right again — you really don't miss. And thank you Don Imus for the opportunity to reach your expansive audience. I was happy to be able to offer much-needed advice to the callers without looking for money or compensation. That's the way it should be when you have a chance to make a difference. It's a great feeling.

One day Don Imus called and asked if I really knew how to cut hair. I said, "Possibly, but what did you have in mind?" He asked if I could come over and give him a haircut, so I said yes and went next door with my scissors. I started to talk about the football game that Brian Levine, my grandson, would be playing in on Saturday afternoon and asked if he and Wyatt would like to come to the game with me. Well, you would have thought I asked him to rob a bank with me. He went on about how cold it was and did I really think that he or his son would go to watch my grandson sit on the bench for two hours. I told Don I was very proud that the Staples High School team in Westport was playing the state championship and recommended that he go, because it was going to be a good game. But he couldn't be persuaded.

So on Saturday, my family and I went to watch the game in Trumbull, CT and not only did Brian's team win, but Brian was one of the heroes of the game. He intercepted a pass in the end zone when the other team was leading 6-0 and ran the ball back over 100 yards. The team won the game and state championship 34-6. The next morning when I went to pick up Larry, I bought 2 sets of all the local papers — one for me and one set for Don Imus. I delivered them to him that morning and pointed out what a great game he had missed. He could hardly believe it. Then when he went on the air on Monday morning, he told the whole story (including the haircut) to his sidekick, Charles McCord, and the whole world. I sure got a lot of calls that week, and was a happy and proud Pop.

The Imus family opened many doors for me, and I met so many wonderful people through Don and his on-air mentions. For instance, Richard Grasso, the former Chairman of the New York Stock Exchange and his wife Lorraine, who took me as his guest to a dinner in downtown NYC with the Congressional Medal of Honor Winners. Talk about champions of our country. I am glad I'm a veteran, although I never had to go to war, but these champions made sure our freedom was protected. They are the true nobility of our country.

Imus also introduced me to a champion of champions, David Jurist, and his wife Alice, who started "Tomorrow's Children Fund" at the Hackensack Children's Hospital in New Jersey and opened their magnificent home to me and hundreds of other people, all in the name of helping others. The Jurists and their wonderful family hosted a wonderful charity event at their house to benefit children. I attended with my son Larry and some of my grandchildren. David is still a great personal friend of mine today and we speak almost every Sunday morning when he speaks to Larry with love and patience. I love you David and Alice. You are the special people God has made a place for. David introduced me to Bobby Thompson, who hit the famous home run against the Brooklyn Dodgers. Bobby was kind enough to sign some balls for me to use in raising money for one of my charities, mainly the Pro Sports Challenge.

Some other connections I made through the Imus family include: Charles & Connie McCord, Bernard, Lou, the Coleman Family (Dierdre's Mom and Dad), Rob Bartlett, Bernadette Castro, her daughter Terri and, of course, the infamous Bo Dietl, former NYC police officer turned security entrepreneur and regular guest on Imus' show, and many others.

> **Mini-Lesson:** *You can never meet or know too many good people.*

Through the Imus', I also met President Jimmy Carter's former Chief of Staff, Hamilton Jordan, who spent several nights in our home while doing outstanding work building the children's charity Camp Sunshine. I even took Hamilton over to New Jersey to show him our High Speed Video operation. He was so impressed that he told Don. Don would sometimes broadcast his show from the Imus Ranch, a working cattle ranch for kids with cancer, 65 miles out in the desert of Ribera, NM. When he mentioned that he wanted to be able to seamlessly see and hear his on-air partners and staff whenever he was at the ranch, I was happy to help by using the 2-way video system technology provided by my High Speed Video Company (HSV), which we provided at our cost.

After a telephone circuit was made available for HSV from the ranch to the production studio in Astoria, NY, Joe, one of HSV's engineers traveled to Ribera with the required hardware and performed the installation at the ranch's studio. Simultaneously, we sent our engineers to the facility in New York, which is headed up by my partner Mike

Maresca. The equipment was installed and the system was tested. The quality of video communication between the 2 locations was spectacular and it all worked perfectly. (Imagine if it didn't. He never would've let me live it down). Many thanks to my partner in the business, Mike Maresca, and Joe, the technical expert, for making it happen for Don Imus.

Soon after, I visited the ranch as a guest of Don and Dierdre to check that the installation was properly in place and was happy to see that HSV system was still working flawlessly with crystal-clear video quality. While at the ranch, I observed the wonderful treatment that the Imus Family gave to the children. The Ranch is immaculate and offers a ton of stuff for both the children with cancer and their siblings to do. The care they get is top notch, and the activities are fun and healthy. They get to ride horses, enjoy nature and have wonderful, healthful (vegetarian) food. Deirdre and Don share their food and their love. As I watched and took pictures, it was enlightening and I wished that everyone were able to help children to this degree. They've really done a great job.

God bless you both for the work you do. I enjoyed your hospitality and loved the interchange we had together with the children. It was obvious that they loved the chance to be on a ranch and have a fun week away. I made an album for my memory bank and was happy to see that the donations I had made were going to a great cause. I even tried to help several of the children get the right doctors and treatment in Little Rock. I especially remember the love you showed to one young man by the name of Davin, a brain tumor patient whose Mom couldn't handle it alone. Don and Deirdre were both begging and pleading with his doctors and the hospital to help Davin.

We called down to Arkansas and had Dr. James Suen and his staff on the ready while Don and Deirdre arranged with NetJet to fly him there. We also got the Guest House Inn to comp his stay while the doctors tried to save his life. Although we tried, sadly Davin didn't make it. In a lovely letter from Deirdre, she thanked me for all of my help and support and acknowledged that we tried together to make a difference in these children's lives. I will always treasure the sentiment. You are a very special lady who is capable of making things happen.

> **Mini-Lesson:** *You can see how relationships intertwine and everyone goes into the same mode, when it's about helping others. I think it's a beautiful thing to witness. Friends are always available to help no matter how big or small the problem. It was about trying to save a life.*

Author and children's health advocate, Deirdre Imus continues to raise her beloved son and fight the good fight for children everywhere. She's also a talented writer who wrote a wonderful cookbook as well as a lifestyle book on "green living." As for Deirdre's grumpy husband, the shock jock and philanthropist Don Imus is still on the radio and television's Fox Business Network doing his thing and courting controversy with his inimitable style and humor. Don, you can play the grouchy old cowboy routine, but under it all you are quite a man with your Lady Deirdre. You've come a long way, Cowboy.

I will always have a deep respect for the Imus family and the love and generosity they've bestowed on others, especially the kids at the ranch. When Don announced that he was suffering from prostate cancer, my heart went out to him and his lovely family. My thoughts and prayers are with him as he receives treatment and goes through the battle I know so well. Get well, Imus. Please call me if you want to start taking the "sea puke" (as you like to call TBL-12/Sea Cucumber Dietary Food Supplement) again, and I'll send it right over — the first shipment will be my treat. The friends I made through knowing you changed my life forever, so I owe you at least a few pages in this book. I'm so glad that the Radar moved next door and I'm constantly amazed at how it allowed me to do so much good for so many others. Everything I learned living next door to a legend like Don Imus was a life experience. Going to his ranch and watching both him and Dierdre doing whatever they could to help children with cancer was an incredible opportunity. As I've said, if you have the chance to do good for someone that needs it, the feeling is great. Just ask the Imus's. Bashert! (God's will).

Long Lost Cousins

My great-grandfather on my Dad's side, had 18 children, so when I was a young boy growing up, I always had many cousins around. It was great. I always made fun of the fact that I had a grandfather named Sam the Rabbi and an uncle, his brother, named Sam the Glazer. I would say that my great-grandparents forgot they had used the name Sam already on another kid, so they named the last one Sam 2. Sam 2 owned Glen Cove Glazing, Port Washington House of Glass, Westbury Glazing, and many other businesses. Many of the uncles became successful and had children, but for some reason or other, I very rarely met most of them, so no relationships were formed. Somewhere I have an entire family of Gershons related by blood and I have no idea who or where they are. Maybe one day we'll reconnect, who knows? In Washington DC however, I have Barbara Silver and her mom, Carrie Silver, and cousin, Jerry Stollman. We keep in touch mostly through email.

Then there is my mother's side of the family. Every Sunday was Family Day, and we all got to see each other. We were so very close growing up and kept the Family Sundays tradition going for years. When my mother's sister Bea and her husband Uncle Oscar (Unk) Fine drove across the country to try to make a life for their family in California, my cousin Ira stayed with us at our house while his parents set things up. Ira was 6 then and he became my kid brother — we would share a bed and sleep back to back. He was 4 years my junior and was my responsibility to walk to and from school. I loved Ira then and now.

Although he moved to California to be with his parents at age 6, we still see each other as often as we can. He's built a very successful life with his wife Barbara and their great family, and we've kept in close touch. We talk two to three times a week (or more). Actually, as I am writing this, I'm on a plane returning from Ira and Barbara's 50th Anniversary party in Los Angeles. Thanks, Ira — I love our brotherhood, and I continue to cherish our relationship. I also have great memories of those wonderful trips we all took together. You taught us about the benefits of cruise ship travel—unpack once and go to many places. What a great lesson learned. Thanks again.

> **Mini-Lesson:** *I personally think that cruise ships offer a great way to travel. They go to many places and offer great rooms, impeccable service, tons of food and exciting shows. Thanks Celebrity and Princess Cruise Lines. Cruising is a great way to make new friends and network with people from all over the world.*

My mother's brother (Al Butler) had a daughter named Elaine (Elaine Butler Jerrold), also known as Cousin Inky. Inky is like my sister. The story goes that I had a hard time saying Elaine when I was a young boy, so I called her Inky (which I guess sounded like Elaine to my young ears). And that's what she's been known as ever since. Inky and I have always been kindred spirits — we were born 364 days apart (she's a year older) and we would share a birthday celebration as kids. We would have a lot of laughs at family gatherings and of course, the mandatory music lessons at Aunt Syd and Uncle Charlie's. Cousin Inky and I lost contact as we got older, but I was very happy to rekindle our bond in later years. After too many years out of touch, we are now back in each other's lives, connected forever by our bloodline and the shared memories of our childhood filled with remarkable relatives. Inky had a long and impressive career as head nurse at Mt. Sinai and married an ophthalmologist named Gerald (Skip), who is a great guy and has a great family.

Through the years, Inky has been a regular visitor to my Connecticut home, taking the train from New York with her daughter Stacy and grandsons. I love when they visit, and we always try to squeeze in a rousing game of ping pong when they're here. It's striking how much the family resemblance carries into generations as Ethan looks so much like his great-great grandfather, my "Pop," David Butler. It warms my heart when I look at him. Inky and I see each other in New York City when I am down there, and we often celebrate our birthdays together with a Carvel cake on which I inscribe "Happy Birthday to Us!" She has been a great to help me in putting together this book, and has given me much love and support during the process. It's been so much fun sharing our memories. I so cherish my cousin and friend and love having her in my life. Thanks, Ink. I love you!

I also have cousins Jackie and Ralph in L.A. whom I try to see on my visits to the West Coast. Ralph Lasher worked with Ira's brother, Jerry helping me run Amtax California when I had the Amtax Equipment Leasing business and they did a great job. I have a few other cousins that I've been close to over the years, but this big world keeps pulling us apart and I've unfortunately lost track of many of them, but I'm grateful when new family members appear. I recently got an email from my cousin Myrna who found me on my website (www.mwalterlevine.com), and now lives in Arizona. Hopefully, we'll get the chance to visit with each other some time soon. She has been asking for a visit. I think that I'm one of the luckiest people alive to have been able to keep so many friendships and family relationships alive throughout the years. It takes some effort, but it's so worth it.

> **Mini-Lesson:** *If you really care and value the relationship, you can open new vistas with blood relations. It takes work on all sides, but when it works, it's so worth it.*

Not long ago, I was asked by my son-in-law Greg if I knew anything about the seltzer business. I laughed at the fact that I'd never shared the fact that my Pop (Mom's father) had owned a soda factory. Actually the word factory is a bit questionable because the production was pretty low-tech. Both the Butler sisters' and their two brothers (Al and Abe) worked with their dad, David Butler at Butler Brothers Beverage Company (BBB) of Maspeth, Queens, producing and selling soda and "Good Health Seltzer" for 10 cents a bottle, or 90 cents for a box of 10. The soda factory they operated out of resembled a shack on rollers. There was no automation in the operation. Foot pedals ran the machines, and the crimped caps were put on the bottles by hand.

I worked there during the summers when I was young. It was hard work — making soda, filling seltzer bottles and then carrying them to the 2 trucks Pop had. A man named Eddie drove one truck and Uncle Al drove the other one. I would carry cases of soda and seltzer up and down six-story buildings to customers throughout Brooklyn and Queens. From Brownsville, East Flatbush and Coney Island all the way to Maspeth and the Rockaways. It was a pretty big territory. You get strong quickly — and tired. I think I made a whopping $1.50 for the week. I made more selling clothes pins. But that's what growing up and learning the value of hard work is all about. You do what you gotta do, and I loved working with my Pop. It was nice to see him in action at his place of business. I learned that it can be really nice to work with family. I'm still a proponent of it today and try to do it with my own family as much as possible. My grandfather practiced what he preached and taught me about hard work every day of his life.

> **Mini-Lesson:** *If you have the opportunity to work with family and learn the family business, do it! It will help you in later years by teaching you to have no fear. It is awfully hard to climb the ladder of success with a case of soda or seltzer on your shoulder.*

"Docta" Levine

2002

When Gabe Selig and his dad, Gad came into my life, I was very impressed with their knowledge of the telecommunications industry. They became wonderful resources for me when I entered the high-speed video business and I learned a great deal from them. So, as you could imagine, I was extremely flattered when Dr. Gad Selig asked me to teach a class in entrepreneurship at the University of Bridgeport in Connecticut, where he is a professor and Associate Dean. Although I was a bit nervous, I had no doubt that I was fully qualified to speak to the students, as I had trained many people throughout my varied and numerous careers. From my days in the hairstyling business and creating in-store crowds for Revlon, Buddy Maurice, and John Pierre Cosmetics, to the early years with the Grand Bahama Development Company and through my years in the alarm business, I knew that I had something to share with young, inquiring minds.

> **Mini-Lesson:** *Sharing yourself is an amazing (and risky) experience. You never know how you will be accepted unless you do it. Read their faces. If you're looking into inquiring minds, you'll know.*

My first speech at the university was very rewarding, and I enjoyed every minute of it. I shared my sales training techniques and many of career tales to a class of forty students. I was happy to return when the faculty invited me back to lecture to an even larger class, and I happily went into further detail on my ideas of what it took to succeed in business. The lectures were apparently, quite successful, and to my surprise and excitement, the president of the university contacted me personally to ask me to run my own lecture series. Imagine that. The feeling was indescribable. I saw it as an opportunity to affect the young minds of the future, to touch lives and passions, and to impart hope, inspiration and motivation.

After I became comfortable with the format, I had an idea. Why not invite fellow entrepreneurs and businessmen who had also started from nothing and made something of their lives. I was sure that each one of them had their own special piece of knowledge or advice to share that could help someone else out there. Because of the high caliber of speakers I was able to secure for the series, the university decided to open the lecture series to the public, and soon we had hundreds upon hundreds of attendees. It was a wonderful experience. I thank Gad and God for the blessings this experience brought to me and Gabe Selig for the introduction.

I spent the next two years running sixteen classes, one per month during the school year. I had the best of the best speaking at my classes. Great friends who gave of themselves freely, with not even a thought of being paid. They only wanted the gratification and pleasure of helping others. I was particularly honored that the president of the university, Neil Salonen and his wife Rebecca, came to every class.

<u>2004 - Bridgeport, Connecticut</u>

One day, Bridgeport University President Neil Salonen asked me to be the guest speaker at the Commencement Graduation of 2004. Now of course, I was very used to getting up in front of groups of people and speaking, but I never had an opportunity to speak to 4,300 people at one time. This was the best of the best, but then it got even better. He also told me that they were going to award me with an Honorary Doctorate — the robe, hat and tassel, the whole nine yards. I would be addressing the crowd as Doctor M. Walter Levine. Me, a high school dropout who got my G.E.D. in the Army while in Germany, took a couple of classes for six months in Colorado and sent away for a home study course from the Alexander Hamilton Institute. I was now going to be the commencement speaker at a wonderful university. It was another one of those proud moments when I had to literally pinch myself to make sure it wasn't a dream.

> **Mini-Lesson:** *If I didn't say yes the first time to sharing with one class of students, then this could never have happened. So, the theory here once again is keeping yourself open to opportunities and relationships.*

I moved the tassel from one side to the other and took the podium when I was called. I then asked the audience to please stand up and shake themselves out, as they had been sitting for over an hour, and while they were standing I asked if they would all say three times, "To be enthusiastic, you gotta act enthusiastic! Boy am I enthusiastic!" The first time low, the next louder, and the third time loud enough to take the roof off the Harbor Yard Auditorium. They did it and it was a great moment. Everyone laughed and was grinning and energized when they sat back down. I then proceeded to tell the graduates what I thought they would need to do to go out there and be successful, and how that would mean something different to each of them. I also stressed the need to do right by others and for society.

When I finished the speech, I got a standing ovation. I can't even begin to describe the feelings that were going through me at the time. It was truly a dream come true. I was now officially M. Walter Levine, Ph.D. My friends and family came to support me and celebrate at the after-party they had for me at a country club. Even the rabbi came. I don't know if I've ever been so elated. I am thankful beyond words to my friends and family, especially my wife, Fritzie, for putting it all together and making that day one of the greatest of my life. I never in a million years thought that I would ever be able to call myself a "Docta."

Over the past years, I have been asked to speak at many events, fundraisers and motivational speaking engagements. I enjoy provoking the audience and watching their faces react to some of what I say. It makes me smile inside knowing that I have reached them. I'd like to thank all of the fantastic guest speakers I've had the honor of hosting during my lecture series. These are people with very limited free time, but the opportunity for them to possibly change one life moved them enough to go out of their way and make a conscious effort to share their knowledge with others. Those generous individuals include my friends:

- **Adnan Durrani**, President of Condor Ventures, Inc/partner of the Blue Chip Venture Company. Founder of Vermont Pure Holding, the parent of Crystal Rock bottled water.
- **Ray Joslin**, President & Group Head, Hearst Entertainment & Syndication/Dr VP, The Hearst Corp., ESPN, ESPN2, ESPN NEWS, -Classic Sports Network, Lifetime Television, Lifetime Movie Network, Lifetime Real Women, and A&E Networks, The History Channel, The Biography Channel and The History Channel/Capital Cities/ABC, NBC
- **Stew Leonard, Jr.**, President and CEO of Stew Leonards's Dairy Stores
- **Marc Lasry,** Founder and Managing Partner of Avenue Capital Group
- **Jim Nantz**, Emmy award winning sportscaster and author, known for his affiliation with CBS Sports and recently awarded Sports Caster of the Year

- **Jeff Schwab**, Intellectual Law Attorney, Ableman, Frayne & Schwab/NYC
- **Joe Tacopina**, Criminal Defense Attorney/NYC
- **John Klein**, Chairman/CEO/President - People's Bank
- **Chris Shays**, U.S. House of Representatives, 4th District of CT

I was also honored by the town of Bridgeport with their Good Scout Award, given annually to an individual who embodies the spirit of scouting. In both his business and professional life, the recipient must display integrity and a commitment to serving and helping others. The Good Scout Award recipient must always be an inspiration and example for our youth. I was so very proud to receive acknowledgment for work that brought me such satisfaction. Although I'm not sure just how much of my childhood behavior would have allowed me to qualify to be a Boy Scout back when I was a kid. In any event, it was a great feeling and I continued to enjoy the ride.

> **Mini-Lesson:** *Be persistent and be consistent! Having it all doesn't necessarily mean having it all at once.*

My Fritzie

January 2007 - Westport, Connecticut

Life was good. My family, friends and business ventures kept me happy and challenged. I was extremely grateful for everything that I had. Time with family, the satisfaction of helping others, magnificent trips and parties, as well as the perspective and gratitude to appreciate the simple pleasures. My cup runneth over. Plus, Fritzie and I would be celebrating our 50th wedding anniversary in the upcoming year. Fritzie had spent two years planning a wonderful Celebrity or Princess Cruise for our entire family to celebrate with us. We were taking all eighteen of them as our guests for two weeks on a trip through Italy and the Greek islands. This was a trip that she could literally visualize, and she was beyond excited to have everyone join us for a wonderful and relaxing vacation in the Mediterranean Sea.

But then, at the start of 2007, two days before my 70th birthday, one of the most difficult times in my life began. We had just returned from the beautiful Atlantis Hotel in Paradise Island, Bahamas, owned and operated by my friend, Sol Kerzner. What a great spot. Our entire family had been visiting Paradise Island to celebrate the New Year for many years now, and we always had a great time. Fritzie and the family were busy preparing a surprise for my 70th birthday, just as they had for my 50th and 60th. When we returned to Connecticut on the second of January, Fritzie looked extremely pale. There was absolutely no color in her face. We thought that perhaps she'd caught a cold on the plane, but we soon learned that was not the case.

On January 12th she went to see Dr. Igal Staw, our family doctor and friend for a check-up. After some blood tests, Dr. Staw discovered that she wasn't registering any white blood cells. He instructed her to go straight to the hospital, as he thought she might have leukemia. Fritzie called me at the office while she headed to the hospital. I told her I'd call the rabbi and get a second opinion arranged immediately. The rabbi did his research and quickly called with information and recommendations for us to travel to Texas and ask for a specific doctor.

I called the Anderson Clinic in Houston as soon as I hung up the phone with the rabbi, and they said they'd get back to me. I panicked. I then called my friends in Little Rock, and they told me to get Fritzie to Arkansas immediately. We called the airlines and got an emergency reservation for 6pm that same day. Our wonderful children, Steve, Leslie and Lori drove us to Newark airport for our direct flight to Little Rock, and although we were worried, we knew that no matter what happened we were all in it together and would get through it.

When we arrived in Arkansas at 10:30pm, our friends Dr. James Suen and his wife, Karen, as well as our great friend, Bonnie Jenkins, Chief Nurse Administrator of the Arkansas Cancer Research Center, were there to greet us. James and Bonnie took Fritzie right to the hospital to check her in and begin testing and evaluation, and Karen took me to the hotel to settle in. At midnight, Bonnie called me with some news that shook our world — Fritzie had AML (acute myologenous leukemia). Karen and I rushed to the hospital to meet up with Fritzie, Dr. James and Bonnie. We all just held hands and cried.

> **Mini-Lesson:** *Although it's sometimes tempting, don't shoot the messenger – give him a strong message to take back. We stood together as a family, and that was how we made it through.*

Everything happened so fast. I couldn't believe that we were just in the Bahamas with our entire family, celebrating the New Year, and now, we were facing the same horror that I faced almost twenty years ago — only this time it was my wife. The rabbi gave us a recommendation of treatment, and when we went out to dinner the next night with doctor Bart Barlogie and his wife, Kathy, we shared it with Dr. B. He told us not to worry; Fritzie was in his capable hands. He told us he believed he could get Fritzie well and that he would personally take care of her. He is one of the top doctors in the country specializing in multiple myeloma. We decided to put our trust in him. "Dr. B fixed you, and he will fix me," Fritzie said.

During the next few months, Fritzie was both an in-patient and an out-patient at the hospital. We took our suite at the Guest House Inn, and our good friends, Tom and Judy Adam, and the wonderful staff could not have been more gracious. I would fly in every other week, spending one week in Little Rock and the next back in Connecticut, so that I could see Larry on Sundays twice a month and keep my businesses going. Our granddaughter, Brittney, spent some time taking care of her Gram in Little Rock instead of taking an internship prior to her last semester of college. Britt was our first grandchild and she and Fritzie had a special bond. Britt wanted to spend that time with Fritzie more than anything, and I was so glad that I could help to make that happen.

We continued to pray and I held Fritzie's hand while they gave her blood transfusions, many chemotherapy treatments, cord cell transplants and hundreds of pills to pull her through the cancer. I begged her to take the TBL-12/Sea Cucumber supplement, but she said, "Dr. Bart doesn't want me to take anything but what he prescribes." Despite the fact that I was alive and well seventeen years and clean of all three of my cancers, she refused. Her answer was always the same. Fritzie was very smart but very headstrong. I asked her, "Do the doctors actually tell you what to eat for breakfast, lunch and dinner as well as snacks?" Her answer was always, "No." "So, why don't you take the TBL-12 as a dietary food supplement?" I would ask. Her answer was always, "It worked for you, but...no." We had more than a few arguments about this subject, because I could never understand what harm there could possibly be in her taking it. I had it shipped to our hotel, kept it in the freezer and used it in front of her daily. I thought I could change her mind, but it never happened. She was hell bent on following the exact words of her doctor, who said, "You don't need that food supplement. I'll get you well with the cord cell transplants and the medicine we'll give you." I'm not sure why Fritzie was so stubborn and put all of her faith in the doctor's words. Perhaps it was because she was a radiologist assistant and x-ray technician at one point, and had completely put her trust in traditional science. I don't think I'll ever understand it.

The trip Fritzie dreamed of for so long never happened. She was in and out of the hospital for over six months. Although I tried to stay positive, I was worried that the world we had worked so hard to create together was falling apart. I knew how much she missed her life. Being away from the beautiful home we'd built on the water and her dear family and friends was very tough on her. We wound up spending our 50th Wedding Anniversary (on the 4th of July) at the Guest House Inn of Little Rock. Tom and Judy threw us a small, but lovely party and even invited Dr. James and Karen Suen, Maria Fontaine (wife of Kenny), and another friend who travelled all the way from Connecticut. He had multiple myeloma and had occupied the room next to Fritzie's at the Little Rock Hospital.

Fritzie continued to fight for her life, but she soon needed to be placed in Intensive Care and put on a ventilator to help her breathe. On July 28th, I decided to order a chartered, private ambulance jet plane to take

Fritzie home to our Garden of Eden in Connecticut. Dr. Suen told me that we would need a doctor to accompany her on the trip. "I'm going with you," he said. Fritzie's Little Rock family and friends hugged her goodbye, helped to wrap her in blankets and put her in the ambulance. Many of the hospital's staff members left their posts to say goodbye with many tears and emotions. It was a sad day for our Arkansas family as well as our family.

Dr. Suen and I each held one of her hands for the entire flight, and she smiled when I whispered, "We're going home." Our children were waiting at the Beachside Avenue house when we arrived, smiling and happy to have their Mom and Gram home at last. Every one of her children and grandchildren spent time with her, holding her hand, talking to her, sharing love and praying. Fritzie couldn't speak, but we knew she was listening and her tears flowed. She was home and, by God's hand, her smile lit up the room. We hoped this would be the answer for her. She held Larry's hand, and he began singing, "You Are My Sunshine, My Only Sunshine" which was one of her favorites. I watched this woman who gave her heart and love unconditionally to everyone in the room, those she held closer to her heart than anything in the world. I sat by her side as the family showered her with love and told her how happy they were that she was home. They left for their own homes later that evening and planned to return early the next morning to spend more time with Fritzie. I sat and held her hand and called a few of her friends to come over to the house to say good-bye.

The hardest thing in the world for me to do is nothing, but there was nothing else that could be done. All I could do was watch it happen. Fritzie stopped breathing late that Saturday night. At the end, I just know that she felt the love we all had for her. Dr. Zelkowitz arrived to officially pronounce her deceased. I stayed in the room with her until they took her away. Her pain had stopped and she was now an angel in our hearts.

Fritzie helped so many people in so many ways during her lifetime. She was an incredible human being. There's so much gratitude I feel toward my beloved Fritzie for all the years of love, family and growing together.

Thank you, my fair lady. You are gone but not forgotten. We share thousands of beautiful memories that will live in our hearts always.

> **Mini-Lesson:** *Family values will guide you and get you through the tough times. I believe that our life together of 50 years has created memories that will last longer than our lifetime. Thank you, Fritzie.*

August 2007 - Westport, Connecticut

We began the difficult task of arranging my wife and best friend's funeral. Bill M., a dear friend of hers, probably her closest friend in the world, asked if he could help with the arrangements. Bill sat next to Fritzie for more than twenty years at AA meetings, and he often told her that she'd saved his life. Because of AA's policy of anonymity, I won't use his last name, but he delivered a beautiful eulogy to the 770 attendees at Fritzie's funeral. He told the crowd how much he valued her friendship and looked forward to seeing her at each meeting. They both also sat on the AA Council. He shared the effect Fritzie had on his life and sobriety with eloquence and poignancy. Bill recently told me that Fritzie is still mentioned and thought of daily at her local AA chapter. Pastor John Danner, from Saugatuck Congregational Church in Westport, gave a very personal service, speaking in detail about Fritzie's life including her humble beginnings, when she was forced to leave home at an early age to work for room and board as a housekeeper and nanny.

He quoted the Serenity Prayer and talked about all of her community service and her devotion to family and friends. He shared with everyone her love of swans, books on tape and flowers, and finally, he asked everyone to honor her memory by living with grace and generosity and compassion. Bill had arranged for Terry Eldh, a Broadway singer who has appeared in numerous shows including Phantom of the Opera to sing "You'll Never Walk Alone" and "Over the Rainbow." As her beautiful voice rang out over the room, there was not a dry eye in the house — there just weren't enough tissues. After the service, we went to the burial ground where hundreds of people joined us. The police told me in Westport that it took hours to get traffic back to normal.

Larry especially missed Fritzie. He was constantly asking everyone, "Where's Mom?" It was heartbreaking. I'm sure I wouldn't have gotten through the day without my family's strength and support. I don't think that at any time in my life I've witnessed such an amazing force of love and strength from my children and grandchildren. They spoke of their mother and Gram with love, compassion and passion, proving so clearly and powerfully to all in attendance that the role Fritzie held most dear in her life, that of being a mother and family matriarch , was a job she excelled at. Bravo, my children! Bravo, Fritzie! As sad as we all felt, as surreal as the scene was in many ways, we made it a beautiful celebration of Fritzie's life. It was well earned.

The first months were very difficult. Every day I would come home to an empty house, full of sadness, tears and memories of Fritzie. I continued to feel her presence throughout the house. After three months or so, I decided that it was probably best to sell the Beachside Avenue home that we loved so much and make a fresh start in a new house. Since I lived in the Westport area for twenty-five years, I wanted to remain in the area, close to my family as well as my friends, who are like family to me. Moving away from Beachside Avenue was a great loss in many ways, but I thought it was the right thing to do.

I was very lucky to find a beautiful home on Sasco Hill Road in Fairfield, CT. It has a huge office where I meet with clients, vendors, business partners, potential investors and most importantly cancer patients. It's where I try to give them hope — whether that means directing them to the right doctor for their disease, or giving them information on the TBL-12/Sea Cucumber supplement and getting positive results with successful medical trials. I am currently involved in a half-dozen different companies that keep my days very full. I try to help others daily with TBL-12/Sea Cucumber and many of my other businesses including the AtmosAir (Green Air Company), High Speed Video, Pill Station, etc., which gives me the satisfaction of making a positive difference in people's lives.

My Pride and Joy

Fritzie and I came from different religious backgrounds and we made the decision to bring up our children spiritually, meaning we gave them love, respect and an example of how to treat others. We wanted them to form their own opinions and make their own choices about spirituality. I'm sure our families hoped for more, but when I look at the result of our decision, it's remarkable and gratifying. I love my family.

I don't believe it's possible to love the children God has blessed me with more than I do. When our 8 pound, 6 ounce firstborn Steve arrived, he had a breathing problem and was placed in an incubator. I'll never forget seeing what appeared to be our giant son Steve surrounded by tiny premature babies in the natal unit. He soon grew strong and happy and gave all he had to his family. I can still feel the pride I had when he was going to his first day of school in Monticello, New York. He adjusted so well to a new town and continued to make new friends. When Steve became a big brother to Larry, none of us fully realized the challenges it would bring for all of us. Because of Larry's special needs, so much of our attention and passion was focused on him when the other kids were growing up. Steve selflessly made many adjustments, and personally took on the role of helper, protector, teacher, playmate and friend to Larry. He anticipated his needs, heard his unspoken voice and got him what he needed at the moment he needed it, just as Leslie and Lori did when they got older.

Steve loved sports — baseball, football and basketball. As I mentioned, he became a 3-letter man in high school. The thrill I got from watching those many wonderful moments from Little League through college ball still fills me with pride. If you're fortunate enough to have a child who participates in any form of school activity, take my advice and don't miss it. Go, enjoy, watch closely, be proud of your kids and show them that you are. You'll be creating magic and memories.

I could never have predicted the great success that Steve would have both in business and in family. He has exceeded my expectations in so many ways, and just as he tried to watch and protect his brother from the possible cruelty that other children can inflict on those who aren't normal and can't defend themselves, he continues to try to help and protect those less fortunate than himself. Steve is a valued member of the community and he and his family have many long standing friendships. They should also be very proud to have helped create the Pro Sports Challenge that benefits all the special children at Lower Fairfield Regional Center (LFRC).

Just as my sons are my pride and passion, my daughters are my heart and soul. My daughters, "The Twins," as we always called them, are identical in so many ways besides their looks. No one except Fritzie and I could tell them apart, and even we had a problem doing so when their backs were turned. In the early years, they loved running around the house, and were always dressed perfectly and identically. They were together constantly and are still best friends. My daughter, Leslie, who is two minutes older than Lori, was always treated as the "Big Sis." It's funny how roles within a family structure are shaped, almost from birth. I remember when they graduated high school and were heading for college in New England, Fritzie and I were so happy to give them a surprise reward for their years of selflessness and devotion to our family and Larry: black and white convertibles. Boy did those girls love those cars.

The Twins have tremendous insight into my soul and they own my heart. In fact, they were, and still are, the heart and soul of the family, never complaining and always smiling — well, almost always. (Just kidding girls). Whether it is helping to care for Larry or handling family tasks, they do so with kindness, compassion and service to others. They've developed true friendships, and have earned respect as involved and caring members of the community. They've made me so incredibly proud. Their similarity to their beautiful mother is a lovely thing for me to witness. Now known as Leslie Oxfeld and Lori Esposito, my Twins continue to watch over me and love me like no one else. In the words of Maurice Chevalier, "Thank heaven for little girls."

Coming from the streets of Brooklyn with nothing and reaching many milestones and proud moments with my family along the way has made me question, each time, "Could it get any better?" The answer was always, "Yes!" My grandchildren — all seven of them — Britt, Sara, Brian, Jamie, Andrew, Julie and Nikki are certainly proof of that. The joy that they've given was something I never even anticipated. They are my legacy and I wish them all the best that life has to offer. I always tell them that if they dream about something that they believe will make them happy, do it with all the passion and love that you have inside of you, and don't think about the money. Do it because you want to and because you can, and the money will follow. Be happy and help others. I hope that these are words that my family and dear ones will always take to heart. So, when they look at themselves in the mirror they can smile and say, "I did it my-self, and I helped people." The reward is a great feeling – something that money can't buy. Try it, you'll love it!

Sundays with Larry

"Life is like a box of chocolates. You never know what you're gonna get."
— Forrest Gump's mother

I believe that my son Larry has been a blessing in all of our lives. I say that even though for years I held on to the fantasy that one day he'd wake up and somehow, magically be…"normal." That he'd whisper in my ear, "How did you like that act, Dad? I sure had you all fooled, didn't I?" And I say with all honesty and some embarrassment, that I would trade everything I own or ever will own for the chance for Larry to be "normal." That being said, I also recognize what a gift he's been. Larry, our lifelong baby, our "love child," who as Fritzie would so poignantly say, "will never graduate kindergarten," has brought our family closer than most. He asks for nothing and gives only pure love and unfiltered emotion. He is our angel here on earth.

Our pursuit of the best treatment possible for Larry has led us from New York to Colorado and back, and then to Connecticut with many detours along the way. But throughout that journey, we've met many wonderful people from diverse walks of life and developed amazing friendships that have enriched our lives in countless ways. In fact, Larry has either directly or indirectly been responsible for our entire family working for charity and giving back to others in one way or another, specifically, the ongoing time and money that we willingly devote to the special children, and because of the work we do for others, I believe that we have been blessed many times over. The mutual pursuit of coming to the aid of our fellow human beings is a very powerful bond.

Larry is the most loving kid in the world, and we love him up to the sky and over the moon. Our life is never dull when he is around. For the last many years, Sundays with Larry have been a constant and cherished part of my life. I drive the 30 minutes to pick him up early in the morning so we can spend as much father and son time together as possible. Upon my arrival at the center, the world's friendliest staff awaits me, shaking my hand and giving me hugs. My son is always dressed and ready to jump in my car and go for a ride – his favorite thing to do in the world. He gives me a big hug and a kiss and says goodbye to his buddies and tells the staff members to "Have a great day!" Many of my Christian friends attend religious services on Sunday mornings. Well, my Sunday morning routine at the center is my form of church. It feeds my soul. I am able to share in the lives of the other men and women who live there, some extremely disabled, and yet so very joyful and loving. It really puts things into the proper perspective.

We head first to the gas station to fill up the tank. Then to the car wash, which Larry loves to watch in action. Luckily, he stopped opening the window while going thru the wash after getting soaked one time. When it happened, I laughed so hard, I cried. Then it's off to Stew Leonard's fantastic supermarket, where we are greeted like family. "Stew's," as most Fairfield and Westchester county residents fondly refer to it, is a very unique place. So unique, in fact, that it's been named in Ripley's Believe It or Not as the largest dairy market in the world. It has a huge selection of the freshest meats, produce, baked goods and, of course, dairy products, at unbelievably low prices.

The sprawling layout covers the length of a football field (or two or three), and snakes through the various departments where the actual production of its wares are showcased to reinforce how fresh it all is. Plus there are lots of little puppet shows, singing stuffed animals and, of course, samples to keep both kids and kids at heart alike, entertained and satisfied. Fortune Magazine named it one of the best places to work in America. Stew Sr. came from a family of dairy farmers and built the business from nothing. My kind of guy. And I've known his son, Stew Leonard Jr., who now runs the day to day operations, for over thirty-five years. I remember when he was just a kid, working for his dad at the store and learning the business from the ground up. He's an amazing man as well and has shown tremendous generosity and support to Larry and the center for many years now, as well as many other charities, too numerous to list.

Every Sunday morning, Larry and I are often some of the first customers there, and we always get a big hug and kiss from Stew Jr. Each week, Larry is equally excited to push the cart from beginning to end of the store as we fill up the basket with a variety of foods, treats and staples. We are greeted with smiles and waves by all of the familiar employees and many of the Sunday morning regular customers — sometimes even some hugs. One time Larry planted a big kiss on the lips of a lady shopper he didn't even know. He mistook her for a regular staff member and wanted to show his affection. Oh my God! The lady naturally thought he was some Romeo who was being fresh and turned red as a beet. I held my breath for a moment, thinking that she might slap him, then quickly jumped in and explained to her Larry's condition. Her face immediately softened and she hugged him. It actually turned out to be a very sweet moment. Funny the way things happen.

Thank you, Stew, and every member of the Stew Leonard family and family of employees as well. You all really take the "How Can I Help You?" principle to heart in your tireless pursuit of customer satisfaction and beyond. I was fortunate enough to convince Stew Jr. to be a guest speaker at one of my lectures at the University of Bridgeport. He packed in a standing-room-only crowd and shared some very entertaining and informative stories of the family business and its very entrepreneurial philosophies, which all start and end with the idea of treating people (most importantly, customers and employees) the way you would want to be treated. The Stew Leonard philosophy is plastered all over his stores: "Rule 1 - The Customer is Always right. Rule 2 — If the Customer is wrong, go back to Rule 1." It's a winning formula. I recently returned from a cruise to the Caribbean, and during our stop-over in St. Maarten, I got to visit with Mr. and Mrs. Stew Sr. and Marianne Leonard, who live there during the winter. They are great people with hearts of gold, and have taken us in as family. Thank you Stew for writing a book about your life. It's an amazing, inspiring story that would make a fantastic movie.

After Larry and I finish up at Stew Leonard's, we continue our Sunday morning routine, usually heading to CVS Pharmacy or Walgreens to pick up a few things we need, or just to walk the store so Larry has something to do. We then visit the Village bagel shop, where Larry again says hello to all of his bagel friends, we load up on the variety of delicious bagels and spreads and head back to my home to fix breakfast and make our weekly phone calls. Every week, dear friends and family members are called so that Larry can say hello and tell them, "I love you. Have a great day!" So thanks, cousins Ira and Barbara Fine in Los Angeles, David & Alice Jurist in New Jersey, Stu & Valerie Gordon in Washington, D.C., Marcia & Don Siegelaub in Westport, James & Karen Suen in Little Rock, Uncle Bob Soll in Florida, and Judy Trupin (Aunt Judy) in Florida. Without all of you at the other end of the phone, our Sundays would not be complete. Larry loves to talk to them and likes to tell them it's raining outside (even when it isn't). He says whatever comes to his mind at the moment. It's fun to watch.

After our phone calls, we often check out a ballgame on television or watch a movie. Sometimes we'll go out for lunch, and other times we'll just stay home to have a meal or sit outside when the weather's nice. In the summer we go swimming in the pool. When Steve and his family or the twins and their families are free, they stop by to visit and Larry is always thrilled to see them almost every Sunday if we get lucky. We get lucky often, and often times we're blessed to have friends stop by for a visit.

Now that Fritzie's gone, I have a wonderful gentleman by the name of Greggy, as Larry calls him who helps take care of Larry's personal needs when he is not at the center and is with me. Although Larry is a man of almost 50 years old, he is of a child's mind and body, so he often has "accidents" when he can't make it to the bathroom in time. Greggy is a caring and patient soul, and having him around has been a Godsend. I realize that I'm very lucky to have someone who takes care of Larry in that way, and I'm very grateful. It allows Larry and the family to spend our precious time together filled with fun, gladness, love and songs.

Speaking of songs, Larry loves music, and the joy and laughter that we all share when we sing along with Larry to the songs he knows by heart is heart-warming. God Bless America, Michael Row the Boat Ashore and If You're Happy and You Know It, Clap Your Hands are all part of his repertoire. Many times, one of the children or grandchildren takes Larry back to Norwalk, stopping at Wendy's or for a hot dog on the way. Larry loves his Sunday routine. The regularity of it makes him feel comfortable and safe, and spending time with family and friends makes him feel loved. Larry is grateful to all of you, and although he can't tell you himself, I think you all know that.

I posed this question to Larry's siblings once: If you had been born as Larry was, what would you want me to do, and how would you want to be treated? Their response was obvious — family loyalty and love is our responsibility and our joy. Larry, we hope you know how very much we love and cherish you. Mommy is watching over you from Heaven. Thanks for being our special angel.

As anyone who knows me can tell you Steve, Larry, Leslie and Lori are my pride, passion, heart and soul. We've been able to create a very close connection, and I feel so blessed to have my children and grandchildren living nearby. Spending time with them is always the highlight of my life. I know that I am a very lucky man. Larry and the other men and women at the center are now called "physically and mentally challenged" (since using the word retarded is no longer politically correct). But no matter what you call it, Larry and his friends at the Lower Fairfield Regional

Center need constant care, 24 hours a day, 7 days a week. Knowing that he has his brother and sisters, as well as the magnificent staff at the center, to look after him with love and kind attention gives me a sense of relief, for which I am so very grateful. Thank you my LFCRC family for all your hard work and love for the children you take care of daily–from the Commissioner to all of the beautiful people who have taken on a mission of care, loyalty, and friendship for one and all.

The Good Life

"It's faith in something and enthusiasm for something that makes a life worth living."
- Oliver Wendell Holmes (American physician, teacher and author)

My morning exercise routine is an important part of my life. I start every day (except Sunday) at 5:55 a.m. with a climb up the steps up to my third floor home gym. I throw on my 3-pound sneakers, grab some weights and walk on my treadmill while watching Don Imus and the news on television. It's an enjoyable and energizing workout that has built up strength in my legs and increased my cardiovascular stamina, all while I learn about the latest happenings around the world. This discipline and routine is second nature to me since my Army days, and it's a great feeling to see the results of my efforts in great muscle tone and greater endurance. If you haven't made exercise a priority in your life, please do. Your body will appreciate it.

Tennis was always a passion of mine, and I was a pretty good tennis player in my day, often beating younger, more experienced players. It felt great. Though I'm not playing much tennis anymore due to a crushed vertebrae and missing discs that came with the Multiple Myeloma cancer, I do enjoy playing golf with my buddies, Don Siegelaub, Dick Corbin, Joe Sweedler, Lenny Rummo, Bob Russell, Bob Soll, Eddie Stravitz and Stew Leonard Jr. Whoever's around and ready to hit the links with me is guaranteed to spend the day laughing and having fun. Ever since Fritzie gave me a gift of golf lessons several years ago, I've had a good time, enjoying the nice weather and company of friends, participating in tournaments and being outside. To me, it's not about the score. In fact, I don't know why I even bother keeping score, really. I look at it this way: If I show up on the links, I done good.

The Man in the Mirror

I've always believed in the power of hard work coupled with the concept of dressing for success, good grooming and looking as professional as possible. Those who know me know that I'm not only a workaholic but a clothes nut as well. My appearance has always been a top priority, starting from early in my career as a hair stylist at the prestigious Fontainebleau Hotel in Miami Beach. Buddy Maurice instructed his staff to always show up for work in proper attire. The male stylists were required to wear nice pressed slacks, a shirt and tie or an ascot to cover their necks and a sports jacket. I followed that rule for years. The women were told to wear a skirt and blouse or a dress. Professional attire was mandatory at all times.

It became a habit for me to dress for success in every position I've held ever since – even on days when I worked alone in my office, and let's not forget about my encounter with Charles Revson in the elevator at Revlon, who sent me home because I was wearing a sweater to work. Needless to say, it never happened again. During my Bahamas years, I dressed in "professional" Bahamian garb, which consisted of a short-sleeved, collared, shirt and pressed pants to take prospective buyers on tours of the island. In the evenings, for dinners out with potential clients or investors, I would always wear a shirt and tie and sports jacket. And when I was knocking on front doors during the years I was building the alarm company, one would never find me without a crisp shirt, suit and tie, even on a swelteringly hot day.

As my income increased, I switched to higher-quality clothing, such as French cuff shirts and cufflinks. Hard work has always brought me tremendous satisfaction and success, but I believe that is only part of the equation. Dressing well and impeccable grooming certainly affects the way others perceive you and, like it or not, it sends a message about you.

It also conveys to others how you see yourself. If you don't take yourself and your appearance seriously, why would anyone else? Even on a tight budget, this goal is achievable with a bit of care and savvy shopping. I highly recommend paying close attention to detail in your wardrobe, grooming and style departments. Along with tenacity, passion, focus and hard work, they are key ingredients to building your career and your life onward and upward. Thank you to the Mitchell Family in Westport, CT for standing by the Levines. Their stores (Mitchell's and Richards) always kept me well-dressed.

Got a Pen?

Here's a little tip that often puts a smile on people's faces. Always have a nice, thin pen on you. After way too many frustrating moments when I've missed a phone number, a name or directions, and once maybe even resulting in a lost sale, I decided to treat myself to a silver Tiffany pen that I carry with me in a small, soft leather case at all times. Ever since, part of my daily attire, tucked inside my sock, is the leather case containing the beautiful pen as well as a small pair of reading glasses. I cannot tell you how good it feels to come to the rescue of someone in a jam with something as simple as a pen at the ready. I've probably helped hundreds of people throughout the years on the street, in restaurants, waiting in line, sitting at an airport, standing by a phone booth, etc. So many feel-good moments, all thanks to my pen!

Life is as good as you make it. I believe that we are all responsible for each other and part of the reason God put us here is to try to help as many people as we can. It's not about the money. It's about doing something nice for someone else – for its own sake. And sometimes, that something can be as simple as replying to the question "Do you have a pen?" with a knowing smile and an enthusiastic "Yes, I most certainly do, and you may borrow it."

I Did It My Way

"No man is a true believer unless he desireth for his brother that which he desireth for himself."
— Muhammad

When I was younger, I enjoyed listening to the likes of Tony Bennett, Frank Sinatra, Dean Martin, Steve Lawrence, Bobby Darin and Neil Diamond. They were champions of entertainment who inspired and uplifted me. I wanted so very much in my own way to give people the same good vibrations as the crooners that I loved had given me. Singing has always been an enjoyable part of my life, and my voice is still pretty good, if I do say so myself. Although I've always had the unfulfilled fantasy of being a singer and entertainer, I'd like to think that my primary purpose in this world is to use my "voice" to raise money for good causes, help those who are in need, lead people to business success, counsel my children and coach them to fight for themselves as I have done all my life.

My gift, looking back, seems to have always been communicating with people, forming relationships, inspiring, motivating and helping others, all of which has made my life so incredibly blessed. For me, it always comes back to the "How Can I Help You?" principle, which is essentially the "The Golden Rule." Doing unto others as you would have them do unto you ensures that you deliver your best 100%, 100% of the time. If you focus on helping others, whether that's your customer, your friend, your business partner, stranger, etc., not only does it help them, but it will come back to you in spades. Believe me, it never fails. Even if it doesn't turn out exactly how you might want or expect, the thought is what it is all about.

I know that no matter how hard you try, you can't please everybody all of the time, but between you and I, it's worth the try. I want to be known as the man that did it for everybody — or at least tried to. As I go through life, I try my best each day to create laughter and positive energy, whether it's in business or with friends and family. I like to think that there is a basic humanity and integrity in everyone; a caring nature and a need to help others that overrides everything else. I would even argue that it is the essence of what makes us human, and I wholeheartedly believe that it is THE secret to happiness. Treating everyone the way you want to be treated is the foundation of everything that I stand for and something that I've always tried to instill in my children and grandchildren. If it doesn't work, it's not because you didn't try.

As I come to the end of this book, which has taken me over a decade to finish, I cannot stress enough, that there are no shortcuts and no easy answers. You have to go through the muck to come out at the other side. I tell the hundreds of people from around the world who contact me each year looking for help and direction to navigate their illnesses, their businesses or their lives, and now I tell you: You must fight. You must believe. This is the fight for YOUR life — no one else's. So don't leave it up to anyone else. Not your family, your spouse, your friends or your doctor. YOU are responsible. Do as much research as possible. Talk to as many people as you can. Do your homework and find the best treatment for YOU. It's you who makes the difference.

I picked up a book while I was at the airport a while back. It was Larry King's My Remarkable Journey. It's a witty and wonderful read. I could only hope that my book brings readers as many laughs, lessons and entertainment as Larry's does. After reading his book, I realize that he and I have more in common than I ever knew. We come from similar backgrounds and have both pulled ourselves up by the proverbial bootstraps. After reading his book, I feel like I know him well. It made me think about how we all come from different homes, some with troubled backgrounds, and how we could all make a difference, each in our own way, helping others who need it. Larry's an extremely funny man and probably the most talented interviewer in the world. Larry, you truly are The King.

Turning the Page

August 2009 - Fairfield, Connecticut

"All human wisdom is summed up in two words: wait and hope."
— Alexander Dumas

Losing Fritzie changed things dramatically for me. I know that I must move on, as life is for the living, but some days are still very difficult. I do feel lucky to be alive and blessed to awaken each day healthy, happy and surrounded by loved ones, with challenging tasks to take on and plans for the future. Life does go on after adversity, tragedy and loss, but "how" of course, is a matter of attitude. I enthusiastically choose to make each day great with an "attitude of gratitude" and service to others. When faced with hard choices or hopeless feelings, I hope you agree that the mind is all-powerful. It's all about how you choose to look at things, and although we all have bad days, maybe even bad months, the sun always comes out, and a storm will always bring a rainbow — you can count on it. Fritzie would often say, "Always love with all your heart up to sky and over the moon," and I continue to live by that sentiment.

I try to make each day that God has generously granted me precious and wonderful. I keep busy with my work, family and friends, knowing for certain that He (or She) has kept me alive for a reason. I feel tremendous satisfaction consulting with the cancer patients and others who contact me for guidance, and I try to help in whatever way I can. Whether it's getting through the shock of a recent diagnosis or struggling to maintain a positive outlook in the midst of great pain and suffering, I try to help them find the strength within themselves that I know is necessary for them to make it through the darkest days imaginable.

My large family of children and grandchildren all continue to bring me great joy, and although they are busy with their own lives, they continue to make me feel so very loved and cherished. When it comes to my family I am continually reminded that I am beyond blessed. My family of friends show me constant support and love, and I'm so grateful for the blessings their friendships bring. The colleagues and partners from the many business ventures I am involved with are an extension of my family, and we have a blast together planning projects and formulating new business ideas, or just having fun planning tomorrow. It really is a wonderful life.

On the topic of finding love, I'll say just a few words on this newest phase of my life. I was blessed to have Fritzie as my wife for fifty years, so the single life has been rather hard for me to navigate. There are many things in your life that will catch your eye but only a few that will catch your heart. Life moves on with you or without you, and sometimes you need to "turn the page," which means that yesterday is over and it's time to move on. The alternative is to stay stuck. For me, without the dream of tomorrow, today became quite a challenge, so I had no choice but to turn the page.

One day I got a call from Ivan Dochtor (a very dear friend who was also my lawyer in the 80s) who asked me to join him in Las Vegas with some friends. Timing is everything in life. I really wanted to get away and since I had promised a keynote to an organization in Las Vegas, I thought it might be a good time to deliver on it. However, there was one catch — it was the same weekend that I was moving into my new house.

But my wonderful family and friends came to the rescue. They thought that it would be good for me to get away for some much needed rest and relaxation after all that had happened, so they generously volunteered to handle the move while I went to Vegas. Many thanks to my children and their families, as well as Leroy (my third son), and my close friends, Carole and Don Sherman, who were enormously generous with their time and efforts. Carole made sure everything was hand—packed, and not a dish was broken in transit. I could never thank you all enough for helping me transport a lifetime of memories to a new, fresh start and dream.

So with their help, the house taken care of, I was able to go to Vegas. I flew out with Ivan and his friends on a Friday and I was very happy to be there. On our first day, we were having a great time dining and playing dice when an attractive lady caught my eye. She was beautiful and a damn good crap shooter too, but I didn't say anything. Then, on the second day I saw her again. She was at my table, standing right across from me, shooting the dice and having a great roll, so I bet with her and we both had a lucky run. I recall saying something to her during her shooting the dice.

We both went to the window to cash in our chips at the same time, and I took that opportunity to introduce myself. Her name was Diana Lynn, and she had a lovely smile, long blonde hair and kind, sparkling eyes. When I asked if she would like to have a cup of tea with me, she agreed. We sat, talked and sipped our tea for three hours, which absolutely flew by. We had a wonderful time chatting, so I took her card and told her I would give her a call, even though she lived in Ohio and I had no desire to date anyone so far away. I called anyway and we set up another meeting in New York the following week. As crazy as it seems, on that day I knew my heart belonged to Diana Lynn.

We flew back and forth, seeing each other as frequently as we could over the next few months, but we missed each other terribly when we were apart. I finally realized that it was foolish to miss each other so much, and not be together all the time. I told Diana that I was in love with her and asked her to come live with me in Connecticut to spend our lives together. She told me that she was in love with me too, and wanted to be with me full time here in Connecticut. Wow, what a feeling! It felt like my boat was rocking and life had given me another chance. That kind of feeling doesn't go away, and for that I am grateful.

We found that we have a lot in common and have tons of fun together. We both love to travel, go the movies, go out to dinner, golf and spend time with friends, and she actually has more clothes than I do — which is no small feat. The close friends that we hang out with (the Shermans, Sweedlers, Siegelaubs, Nicotras, etc.) and our families have accepted us as a team and we love being with them. We are grateful that my children, grandchildren, her mom, her sisters and her daughter, Summer, are all on our side and want us to be happy. Together we are finding the happiness we have searched for. I am very fortunate to have been able to have a second chance at life with the right person.

When one has to face the prospect of creating a new life after losing a partner I think it's wise to put yourself out there, get involved with people and see what life brings. I believe that life is better when you have someone special there to share it with. If you're lucky enough to find someone you believe is right for you, as the song says, "Once you have found her, never let her go." I've been fortunate to have found a wonderful lady by the name of Diana Lynn to spend my life with. Thanks Diana for your beautiful smile, your sweet ways and your patience. I'm very lucky to have you in my life — you are a ray of sunshine. Besides being very smart you are a great friend and I'm glad we make each other happy — at least most of the time. (Just kidding!). I just made you laugh, didn't I?

From Nuttin' to Something

"Success seems to be connected with action. Successful people keep moving. They make mistakes, but they don't quit."
— Conrad Hilton, American Hotelier

I work wholeheartedly each day on all my various enterprises and projects. Sometimes I can't even keep track of it all. Thanks KB (Kathy Beck) for keeping so many things in order. You're an amazing assistant. I've been called a serial entrepreneur, and I guess that is an apt description. I know I've been called worse things in my life, so that suits me just fine. It's busy and fulfilling, although every once in a while, I yearn for the old days when I ran my clothespin business, went to the movies, drank Coca-Cola, ate candy at Marge's Candy store and hung out with my buddies on the streets of Brooklyn (okay, maybe not). I've worked hard and feel content with my achievements and my life; yet those simple days of having "nuttin" had a special charm all their own. As long as I can remember I wanted to make "something" out of myself, and I am still trying.

I always knew that I was strong-minded, strong-willed and had the capacity to learn and do anything I thought I could. I was extremely lucky to have been born to loving parents, who came from humble beginnings and never discouraged me from pursuing my dreams. I then found a spouse whose tireless support and accommodation enabled me to explore the road less travelled and achieve my full potential. The mind is the most powerful tool in the world. It can beat anything. It enabled me to beat being poor by working harder and longer than most people, and it also allowed me to beat three cancers with those same techniques. And with God's help, I hope to have another thirty or so good years on this earth to find new ways to help more people.

I just returned from New York City after my twice-a-year checkup and all looks very good. I went to see Dr. Jagannath at Mt Sinai Hospital with one of my 10 year friends and fellow Multiple Myeloma survivor buddies, Ken Makowka, who happens to be doing great on the TBL-12/Sea Cucumber. Like me he is an entrepreneur, a believer, and a cancer survivor. We made a pact that we go and come back together. We get our check-ups minutes after each other and laugh through the tests. It helps to have a partner rooting you on. After the check up, Diana and I flew down to the Bahamas for a few days to recuperate from the last several months of hard work (and to play some craps, of course). It was wonderful to get back to my Bahamas where I had so many happy days. It feels good to be alive, and I truly could not ask for more – except maybe to be able to help more people, and hopefully this book will help me do that by sharing my story. If I can inspire just one person to dig deep and find the strength that lives in their core – deep within their bones — I'll consider this book a success. It's there, but remember, it's up to you to find it.

I know that not all cancer patients are as lucky as I am. Many don't have friends and family who are single-mindedly devoted to getting them through their ordeal, and most don't have the monetary resources needed to get the best treatment available. Cancer is no fun, I know that. There's only so much one person can do, I know that too, but I am honored to do whatever I can. While I wish I could do more, what I believe I can do better than most is to inspire others. When people come to me frightened by their diagnosis, or even worse, shocked at the lack of hope their physicians impart to them, they are desperately seeking a motivator to help them survive, thrive and fight for their lives. I want to provide them with the tools to do so. In fact, I consider it my duty to give them the hope and faith they will need to fight with everything they've got. I believe that God wants me to help.

Each and every visit, phone call and email that I receive gives me a sense of purpose. Helping others see that they hold in their own hands the capacity to make each day the greatest day of their life warms my heart and fills me with inspiration. Not a day goes by that I don't feel grateful, spirited and joyful to be alive, healthy and doing what I do. When I look in the mirror I often smile and say to myself, "Damn, how lucky I am." I take great pleasure in all of my business and philanthropic activities, and enjoy such a full, rich life that I'm challenged daily to keep up with. Life is beautiful and so worth living. I'm not saying that everything and every day is perfect, but it is worth the fight to stay alive and make it work better.

I've never written a book before, and let me tell you, it ain't easy. But one thing I learned in the process is that if you don't bare your soul it just doesn't feel right, so I really tried to be as honest as I could in my writing. It was often difficult, but in my opinion it's the only way to be and the only way to move forward, otherwise, why bother, right? As I type these last words and glimpse the finish line, I feel that my life has just begun again in many ways, and I think that writing this book has been a big part of that.

Overall, my life has been a heck of a good ride. When I look back, I feel good about where I am today. Emotionally it's sometimes been very challenging to stay positive and achieve growth daily, but it's worth it. I feel like I've been blessed spiritually by being able to walk with and talk to God as my friend. The lessons learned along the way gave me the strength to share and help others have a better life. If by my intervention, I can help another person, it is my ultimate joy and pleasure. I believe that is the gift that I have been given and freely pass on the gift to you. I live with the belief that my passion of "How Can I Help You" really makes you a better person. Try it. It will work for you too.

I work daily on projects with my right hand KB and look forward to the interchanges we have with patients and others whom we are helping, as well as the never-ending business opportunities that we have fun with (mostly) every day. Our minds are expanded constantly and we never know the potential success that could come from each meeting or phone call. We are grateful to the people that believe in us, the food we share and the fun we make out of each opportunity daily.

Thank you, Virginia for all the hard work deciphering this book, chapter by chapter. If along the way we can make someone smile by sharing an experience that will help them succeed in their daily businesses, motivate them to build more businesses or enable them to tap into their own strength to fight their battle with cancer or some other illness, then we've succeeded. Virginia's guidance and support in the penning of my memoirs has been an immeasurable help and I truly appreciate her sharing her talent on this very personal project.

This has not been the easiest of projects in my life but getting my story and my thoughts down on paper so that people can perhaps relate to it is very fulfilling to me. Life really is what you make it and hopefully you can relate to my story, or share it with a family member or friend that you think would benefit. Life can offer some wonderful opportunities. Even when you think it's the end, it can be a new beginning. As Nike says, "Just do it!" If you believe in yourself, you can do great things. You can beat poor and beat cancer, like I did, or who knows what else you can accomplish? Just look around.

Thank you to the readers who hung in there and read to the end of my musings. I hope you enjoyed taking this trip with me and hanging out for a while. Perhaps my little pieces of insight can be helpful to you in some way. I never forget how blessed I am, and I never take even one day for granted. Have a great day and don't forget to make it count. Finally, please remember to ask on a daily basis (at least) the most important question in business and in life – the simplest path to happiness and success – that's right, all together now – "How Can I Help You?" Learn it, love it, live it — always — and you won't ever be disappointed. I promise.

◼ Life Lesson #11 - God Helps Those Who Help Others:

When I speak with people who are seeking my help and advice, I do it because I can. My time is theirs. It's just one human helping another. In the personal note she sent to me, Mother Teresa asked me to continue to give back and help those who need it. I am honored to do so and will continue to do so until the day I die. Helping others to live better, healthier lives and overcoming the obstacles they face in business, illness and relationships is the ultimate fulfillment for me. It's truly all about sharing and caring, and all stems from passion and compassion.

"God bless us, everyone!"
— Tiny Tim

CHAPTER TWELVE
Parting Thoughts
and Walter's Top 40 Tips on Winning

LIFE LESSON #12...
THERE IS ALWAYS MORE TO LEARN

I know that I've shared some of these nuggets throughout the book, but here are some parting thoughts that I've compiled into a handy list of my Top 40 Thoughts on Winning. I find that they can be a great pick-me-up when you need an instant shot of motivation and inspiration. I suggest you try to pick a different one to focus on every day.

WALTER'S TOP 40 THOUGHTS ON WINNING

1. If you wonder why good ideas go bad, it may start with you. Open your mind!
2. A champion never gives up — are you the best you can be? You'd better be.
3. When you start a journey, ya gotta take some risks.
4. If you have an idea, it's up to you — only you — to make it work. Visualize. Inspire. Think success. Write it down. Have a plan!
5. If it's what you really want, look to yourself to make it happen, but you have to really want it and live it with all your heart. Remember it's about passion.
6. It ain't about the money. It's all about doing something to help someone else. When you come from this place, people will pay you all the money you'll ever need, but it doesn't come for cheap. You have to deliver and earn it by being better than your competition.
7. Attitude is everything! Learn to think like a winner. There's no room for negative thoughts.
8. Admit when you make a mistake. It builds your credibility, but only if you work to correct it. Fix the situation.
9. Think to yourself daily: if I only had a short time to live, what is it that I would want to do, build or be remembered for?
10. Dare to dream big! It takes just as much effort to dream small. It's your choice.
11. Have a sense of humor. I promise, you'll need it.
12. Will you give the best of yourself? You'll need to if you want to win.

13. Pursue your goals with passion. If don't have passion for something, you don't love it enough. Then do something else.

14. Author, Jim Nantz said that the power of his dreams helped to make him the success he is. It also made him the man that he is. He started young. Do it now.

15. You are the only person in the driver's seat and the architect of your life and future. Why not do something great?

16. Give a gift of more than money. Give of yourself and teach integrity. You get what you give.

17. Let God and spirituality into your life so you have a friend to talk to all the time. You're never alone.

18. Do things to help others - it will help your life and bring you closer to God and people.

19. People only buy two things in life: value and benefits.

20. Enthusiasm, like passion, will give you the attitude to eliminate fear and negativity. "To Be Enthusiastic, You Gotta Act Enthusiastic!" Say it often. "Boy, Am I Enthusiastic!"

21. It's not really that bad out there, it's only bad in your head. Change it.

22. Never be a railroad worker – be in the transportation business. Expand your mind. Grow.

23. In new business and all business, listen to what the man or woman says (the customer). When dealing with a potential customer, give them a reason to go with you — then offer and deliver better service than anyone else.

24. Be ethical and maintain your reputation at all times. It'll make the world a nicer place, everywhere you turn and you will get referrals.

25. The world of business is like show business – there's no business like it. Selling, like acting, is connecting to people and having them accept your story. Building relationships is key. Connection is everything.

26. You'd better believe in yourself or no one else will.

27. You can fix the problems in your view. If you can see it, you can make it better. Look. Connect.

28. Lead from trust, not fear – but lead.

29. Desire is stronger than skill. Do it.

30. Leaders get mad. Anger is a part of success. Frustration brings forth change and solutions.

31. Put your energy into constructive actions.

32. Don't lower your standards. Raise the bar. Be true to yourself.

33. You only need one person to make a difference. Be that person. It will change you inside and out.

34. Bouncing back after you fail is the most important key to new success. Keep trying and build again. Ben Franklin said, "I haven't failed….I just found 10,000 ways that don't work."

35. People do business with people they like. What's your style? Smile — be happy.

36. Write letters to people if you read or hear about them and if something about their story inspires you. Tell them.

37. Watch your body language and remember to smile – even when you're on the phone. It comes through over the wires. So put a small mirror next to your phone on your desk and keep an eye on yourself. People will hear "the happy" in your voice.

38. Do the right thing – every day of your life.

39. Give of yourself and show acceptance of everyone you meet. Then watch the magic happen.

40. Sometimes you just need to turn the page.

Life Lesson #12 — There is Always More to Learn:

So let's keep going. Have you been inspired to come up with a few of your own thoughts on winning? If so, jot them down in the margin. If you're ever having a down day and need a little extra something to help you get enthusiastic, come back and reread these and your own pearls of wisdom. And keep adding to them!

The End

(or a new beginning…)

Mr. Walter Levine
P.O. Box 355
Greens Farms, CT 06838

March 1, 2006

Dear Walter,

The whole idea of swallowing "Sea Cucumbers" seemed absolutely appropriate for a man struck with Multiple Myeloma. One as strange as the other. Why not I thought? Food from the sea, where we all began, harvested in ancient Asian waters. Perfect.

It was for me. It gave me hope, a hedge against the modern medicine man should their magic fail. This gift came with the most-determined, relentless, avalanche of caring that I've ever encountered. Who is this guy? And why am I glad he's rooting for me?

Walter, I'll never forget all those calls to my home and to the hospital. They pulled me out of the listless boredom and self-involvement that the cancer creates, and navigated me towards realistic and worthwhile goals. My survival was to mean something to a lot of people, so start to plan you told me. Take the cucumbers and plan.

I took them and took them, and took them. And I did have more energy than my fellow sufferers. I took them and kept my eye on the prize. And I survived. I consider the cucumbers an essential part of my recovery. I'll always be grateful to you, Walter, whether I live two more years or twenty – it doesn't matter. That you were there, matters.

With great affection,

Roy Scheider

Roy Scheider

---

12 ROLLING RIDGE ROAD

GEORGE S. HARKINS
FAIRFIELD, CT 06430

(203) 255-1672

Mr. M. Walter Levine
541 Sasco Hill Road
Southport, Ct. 06824

10/20/08

Dear Walter:

Twenty - five months ago, after a Ct-Scan, I was told I had inoperable pancreatic cancer. One month later (x-ys) I started taking TBL12 (Sea Cucumbers). Since that time I have had close to 70 chemo-treatments, 1½ yrs. of the Tarceva pill, Cyber knife radiation and stents put in my bile duct.

With minor exception I have been able to lead an active life to the dismay of my doctors. They no longer think its funny that I take sea cucumbers as they cannot explain my good health. I am 81 yrs. old, 6'2", weigh 185 lbs., play golf twice a week, swim and travel. I am living each day to the fullest - so far so good. All my best and thanks for getting me on the Sea Cucumbers.

Sincerely
George S. Harkins

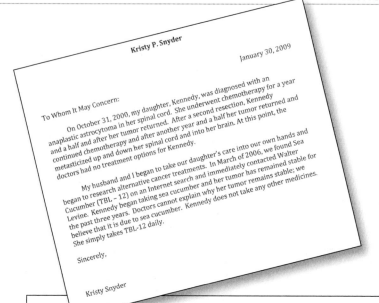

Kristy P. Snyder

January 30, 2009

To Whom It May Concern:

On October 31, 2000, my daughter, Kennedy, was diagnosed with an anaplastic astrocytoma in her spinal cord. She underwent chemotherapy for a year and a half and after her tumor returned. After a second resection, Kennedy continued chemotherapy and after another year and a half her tumor returned and metasticized up and down her spinal cord and into her brain. At this point, the doctors had no treatment options for Kennedy.

My husband and I began to take our daughter's care into our own hands and began to research alternative cancer treatments. In March of 2006, we found Sea Cucumber (TBL – 12) on an Internet search and immediately contacted Walter Levine. Kennedy began taking sea cucumber and her tumor has remained stable for the past three years. Doctors cannot explain why her tumor remains stable; we believe that it is due to sea cucumber. Kennedy does not take any other medicines. She simply takes TBL-12 daily.

Sincerely,

Kristy Snyder

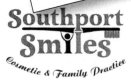

www.SouthportSmiles.com

Dear Mr. Levine,

As you know, I was diagnosed with large B-cell, non-Hodgkin's lymphoma in September 2004. That fateful day, I felt that the days of my life were numbered. I was given an early death sentence with an incurable, fatal blood cancer.

However, the very next day I contacted you to explain my predicament. It was on that day that you put me on the TBL-12 sea cucumber regimen. You showed me the most recent research and testimonials, and gave me the pep talk of my life! You assured me that I was not going to die and must get on with my life.

Walter, as a 46 year old dentist with a thriving practice and father of two beautiful girls, being married for 20 years, this news can hit you like a moving freight train. Despite the love and support of my immediate and extended families, this disease does not care. Additionally, your support and confidence in this trying time has been of utmost comfort. Without your presence and advice, I do not think I would have made it through this most difficult hurdle in my life. I thank you with all my heart.

A year and 2 months have passed! I take the sea cucumber religiously every day without fail. I'd like to share my results from Yale University, where I have been under care for this duration. My beta-2-microglobulins, M-protein levels, white blood cell count, platelets, and hemoglobin and hematocrit have not changed from the day that I was diagnosed! In fact, some of my results over the past year (in which I get tested every 3 months) have gone down. The physicians at Yale don't understand why my disease has not progressed. They have me on a holding pattern, with no treatment necessary. The PET scans and MRI'S of my entire body reveals no tumors!

Mr. Levine, I feel that this incredible sea cucumber has given me a new lease on life. I recommend sea cucumber to every cancer victim that I meet. As a health care provider, I hope that the mainstream medical world will research this amazing supplement and save others!

I will continue to keep you updated with my physical progress. I am indebted to you for prolonging my life.

Sincerely,

Joseph A. Filiero, D.D.S., M.S.
Chief, Restorative Dentistry
St. Barnabas Hospital, N.Y.
Private Practice, Southport, CT.

Walter:

Please see below. This letter was written to friends and family from my wife Denise. Thank you for all of your support and guidance.

Ted Spencer – *Cancer Survivor*

Hello friends and family-

I wanted to take the opportunity to share some good news. Many of you have already heard that Ted has crossed his first big hurdle on this road of recovery. On September 8th he had a full body PET scan to look for any cancer evidence and it was completely negative showing that he remains CANCER FREE!! His radiation oncologist, though very confident in his work, admits that he is even amazed at the progress that Ted has made. He said it really is a small miracle! Ted owes it to TBL12/Sea Cucumber. It has added incredible value to his good health and aided his my speedy recovery. Ted believes that this product should be given to every cancer patient in the world because if it did so well for him it must be able to do great things for other people as well. Walter Levine was introduced to Ted by our very good friend Bob Russell who has watched over him with the care of a parent. I am extremely grateful to both Bob and Walter for making TBL12/Sea Cucumber available to Ted. Thank you from my family and from me. Dr. Son reminds us that the tumor was very significant in the back of Ted's throat and now all he can see is healthy tissue. He can't even tell the difference between the left side where the tumor was and the right side that was not affected. He asked Ted if he could use him as a reference for other patients with a similar diagnosis that are wondering which course of treatment to choose. Ted told Dr. Son he would be happy to share his story and help in any way that he could. From here he will continue to have CT scans every 3 months and as long as those stay clear he is good. If anything new or irregular shows up on a CT scan they will order another PET scan and the cycle will continue for at least the next year and a half. He continues to look amazing and he says he has never felt better physically. He has been working out like crazy and getting back in shape rebuilding some of the muscle mass that he lost in treatment. We do yoga classes together 2-3 times a week and he continues to ride his bike preparing for next year's CT Challenge. This year, as most of you know, he completed the 50 mile bike ride and raised almost $8,000 in 3 weeks for cancer research (thanks to all of your support). It was an amazing event that we both plan to participate in next year. I was so inspired I am trying to do the 50 mile race next summer and he is training to do the 100 mile! We will of course keep you all in the loop with all the details as we get closer. Anyone interested in riding on his team let me know. You have your choice of distances 12 mile, 25 mile, 50 mile or 100mile. In the meantime, he is enjoying his time off (he is on administrative leave until January) and he has been spending a lot of time coaching his own children for a change of pace and they are loving it. We hope you all had a great summer and you are now enjoying this beautiful autumn weather. This is Ted's favorite time of year……

Love-

Denise Spencer

GRIFFEN HEALTH SERVICES CORP.

JOHN BUSTELOS, JR.
PRESIDENT
RETIRED

MR. WALTER LEVINE

DEAR WALTER,

MY WIFE JOAN AND I OWE YOU A DEBT OF GRATITUDE. JOAN WAS DIAGNOSED WITH STAGE 3 BREAST CANCER IN OCTOBER OF 2004.

THANKS TO GOOD MEDICAL CARE, PRAYER AND TBL-12/SEA CUCUMBER, SHE IS FULL OF ENERGY, ENTHUSSIASTIC AND CANCER FREE....NOW A YEAR AND HALF LATER.

WE CAN'T THANK YOU ENOUGH FOR INTRODUCING US TO TBL-12/SEA CUCUMBER.

SINCERELY,

JOHN AND JOAN BUSTELOS

Walter Levine

A brief summary of my relationship with Walter Levine:

About 30 years ago, Walter joined our tennis group in Westport, CT. He was exceptionally friendly and had a great personality. However, he seemed a bit different. For example, he always opened two cans of tennis balls because he wanted to reduce the time and effort of retrieving balls from only one can. Nevertheless, there seemed to be something special about him, but at that time, I could not identify what it was.

A year or so later, I was informed that Walter had been diagnosed with bone cancer. Shortly after that, Walter showed up in a brand new Rolls Royce Corniche convertible.

Several years later, Walter and Fritzie joined another couple with whom we were having dinner. Walter suggested we meet to explore how we might to do some business together. That was it! When we met one-on-one, I had an opportunity to discover the real Walter beyond a flamboyant salesman. That was the beginning of a very extraordinary friendship.

As Walter beat the odds by successfully fighting a diagnosis of terminal cancer, he devotes half of his time helping others who are inflicted with diseases. Walter identified a Rabbi from Israel who spends his time researching and identifying the best doctors to treat specific conditions. This connection enables Walter to recommend the best person for him or her to see. Additionally, Walter believes that a sea cumber derivative is largely responsible his cancer cure. He offers this natural product, at his cost, to patients. I cannot begin to tell you the numerous formerly dying patients, I observed while visiting Walter's office, who are now living normal lives and owe their life to Walter's intervention.

From a business standpoint, Walter is one of a kind. I have been fortunate to be involved in several of Walter's projects. He knows just about everybody and is uncommonly ethical. He wants everyone in a business deal to be a winner. As with ill people, Walter helps everyone, but do not cross him. He has an uncanny instinctive insight into people and is extremely sincere and caring.

I trust Walter completely and would do just about anything to for him. He is truly one of the finest individuals I have ever met.

Sincerely,

Dick Corbin

Monday, March 11, 2002

Dear Walter,

There are really no words to express how I feel about you and the things you have done; for my husband and particularly for Daevin Kirschner. When we had all lost hope you were there to help us. You were remarkable in your enthusiasm, your optimism and your willingness to do everything in your power to save this child's life. You never said no. You answered every call. Boy, that must be some deal you made with God.

Never in my life did I envision begging doctors to help a sick child who was dying. You got us the best doctors in the world. You could not have done more than you did. And when Daevin died, you were there to honor him with your presence and your respect.

Walter, you are my friend. I thank you and I am proud and honored to know you.

Love,

Deit

From Walter's daughter, Leslie Oxfeld...

My dad has taught me many valuable lessons. He has always taught me to have a friend, you must to be a friend. Friendships are one thing my Dad always worked on. He taught me the meaning of commitment and discipline. He taught me to love and reach out and help other people.

My Dad has a heart of gold. He created many long lasting memories. We bonded as a family of 16 on beautiful vacations. We started off with Pizza nights every Friday night. When all the kids schedules got more demanding, we switched to Sunday morning bagels with Larry. The meaning of family was the biggest lesson for me, how important you need to make each day count.

Daughter Lori Esposito

I always loved being the youngest in the family even if it was only by two minutes. I grew up in a family with four children, a workaholic father trying to always provide the very best for his family and a busy mother who was not only an X-Ray technician but a devoted mother to a special needs son. You can say at times our Levine household was hectic! Dad and Mom seemed to make it work! There was not one day that we all didn't feel loved, needed, and cared for. We were always encouraged to have good work ethics and be independent. It was very important to my parents to do charity work and give back to society! We were raised in the best of both worlds with my Dad being Jewish and my mom Catholic. There wishes were to respect everyone and they felt that there was a God big enough for everybody! I graduated High School, graduated college with a degree in Physical Education(Science), and ended up working for the family business at Dictograph Security. Seven years passed, I fell in love with my husband, Ray Esposito, married, had two children, Jamie Rae and Julie Nicole and started my family.

I feel lucky and blessed to have parents that were married 50 years and kept our family together as one. We had our Friday night Pizza nights that included singing and dancing with all the cousins, Dates on Sundays to take all the grandchildren shopping for something special and to this day, we vacation together(thanks to dad) and celebrate life!!! What's better than that???

Granddaughter Brittney Levine

Hi Pop,

Sorry for the delay in my paragraph- I love you!

Being the first-born of seven grandchildren, I have always had a special relationship, rather a deep connection, with my Pop and Gram. My Pop was and is an integral part of my life growing up, making it a point to keep our family together during Friday "Pizza Nights" and family vacations. He has taught me lessons that I continue to practice in my everyday business and in life. Honesty, integrity, and compassion for others are some of those key values. The biggest gift that he ever gave me was when he asked me to stay and take care of my Gram during her final months in Arkansas battling cancer. I owe him everything for giving me that special time with her. I'm so proud that you have finished this goal of yours Pop, and I will always love you up to the sky and continue to carry on the values you have taught me each and every day. -Your #1

"Rarely in a person's life do you have the opportunity to share a unique friendship with someone has special has Walter Levine. Walter is my teacher, my mentor, my golf partner, but most importantly the best friend a person could have with all of Life's ups and downs! Walter's life experiences are unique and "Boy" can Walter spin a life lesson like no other! He is the master of turning very complicated issues into simple life lessons that everyone one can learn from regardless of age. From Brooklyn to the King of the Gold Coast, there is nobody better than Walter. The Legend, My Idol, My Friend, the Great Walter Levine is a must read story for everyone with a love for life !"

Bob Russell
FOW (Friend of Walter's) and caddie at Birchwood

I fondly recall meeting Walter Levine about 2 years ago.

He was "holding court" in the greenhouse of his beautiful oceanside estate, entertaining fast arriving ideas about new inventions, products, business problems.

At times, prompted by a product, he would initiate phone calls to powerful and wealthy friends, who almost always answered immediately.

This activity was going on while Walter wrestled with the imminent death of his beloved wife Fritzie.

At one point, he turned his attention to our invention: a telemedicine based medication adherence system. His questions were quick, deep, thoughtful-he saw both the humanitarian and business values.

Then Walter architected the searching for funding, recruitment of an executive team, sales strategy within 15 minutes.

Walter's surroundings showed the level of his financial prowess and success.

But his approach to my partner and me was inviting, warm, totally without pretense.

He shared his first business success as a child: washing, branding and reselling discarded clothes pins found behind tenements in Brooklyn. This was a brilliant, street smart man!

As I examined photos of Walter with the "rich and famous", my eye was immediately taken by pictures of Walter with Mother Teresa and a letter she had written to him.

Then I learned about his heart: surviving multiple forms of cancer, he had turned his philanthropy to helping others obtain needed or novel treatment.

Caring for a son with Mental Retardation, he and Fritzie found another lifelong cause to support.

Walter recalls the aphorism of Maimonides: If I am not for myself, who will be; if I am only for myself, what kind of man am I?

To Walter with Love,
David Bear, MD
Founder, Senticare, Inc

Grandson Brian Levine

Pop,

Pop is a preacher- he preaches **through experience** about how everyone should love, be caring, optimistic, genuine and passionate. Pop has a deep love connection with his family, business partners and friends—they *are* his life. Pop has a side to him that always puts others first-- The contributions he has made to children with mental retardation and people suffering from cancer are beyond remarkable. I have yet to see someone more optimistic and passionate than my pop. When it comes to work and sales he can flat out sell anything --H e has a grace in his delivery that makes many people want to do business with him. He lives and believes, "If you think you can, you can. If you think you can't, you won't." People will always know one thing about pop – he is a genuine guy who wears his heart on his sleeve. He will fight to live up for his word and integrity.

What does one say to capture the essence of a 45 year relationship. I could write the whole book but I, as a trained (and damned good) lawyer have always believed that less is more, Bullshit fills pages but love and affection and admiration speaks more loudly.

I met you through Mel when you were working for Beauty Industries selling land for that dynamic trio, Mel Harris, Herman Perl and Nick Morley. Mel was my first client in practice and I have represented him for almost 47 years. Don't remind him of that. He'll think he is getting old.☺He is not. He grew up with Valerie starting at age 23. Over those years I, also, at various times represented you and Nick Morley. What whirlwind action concerning those very shy and retiring personalities.☺

`I did not know you as Marvin Hairdresser to the Stars in the Borscht Belt. However, almost twenty years ago my involvement with you took a major increase. You developed Multiple Myeloma. My earliest recollection of that small impediment☺ was of you in New York Hospital near death. I stayed with you on one occasion when you had many hours of major blood purification and remember holding your hand. You really were far braver than I, and Fritzie, who adored you, could not face that. She did, however, stick with you and by your side through thick and thin throughout your repression and stabilization and until her very unfortunate medical problem could not allow her to it any longer. It was then you who stood by her. You are, indeed, the Poster Boy of Arkansas Medical Center and Multiple Myeloma. It did not beat you. You beat it.

This is really a small synopsis of our relationship which also encompassed many, many years of visits to Bluewater Hill and Beachside Avenue with you and Fritzie, who both Valerie and I adored. Never on any occasion, weddings, Bar or Bat Mitzvahs or important anniversaries did either you or Fritzie or Valerie and I not all join together in the occasion. We had very, very happy times and wonderful memories.

In all, my friend, my admiration for you continues to grow, You have helped so many so selflessly that I have no doubt in the future you will meet Mother Theresa in heaven. You never were "nuttin" you always were "somethin" and, hopefully you will be somethin for many, many more years to come.

Valerie joins me in sending you all our love.

Best,   Stu

Life brings with it many happy surprises. Walter first became a client --- then a friend --- and then a member of Barbara's and my extended family. Despite being near death and having to experience the agony of watching a loved one's passing, Walter continues to view each day and the future with the eyes of one holding a half-full glass. I can think of no greater honor than simply to be considered his friend.

Jeffrey A. Schwab
Abelman, Frayne & Schwab

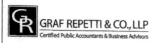

GRAF REPETTI & CO., LLP
Certified Public Accountants & Business Advisors

www.grafrepetti.com

August 14, 2009

In 1940 when I was 5 years old, I moved into 214 Rockaway Parkway, Brooklyn NY
Apt. 1A. My next door neighbor was Marvin (AKA Walter) Levine in Apt 1B.

It seems I couldn't leave the building without a fight with Marvin even though we spent
as much time in each other's apartment as in our own.

If there was ever anyone who was rated most likely to not succeed it was Marvin Levine.
In retrospect the title of his book from "Nuttin to Something" is perfect.

I moved away when I was 16 years old and basically lost contact with Marvin.

About 20 years later I got a call from someone who asked me if I lived in Apt 1A at 214
Rockaway Parkway. I asked if this was Marvin and he said I'm now Walter.

We have maintained our relationship since then for the past 30 years.

I have gained a new respect for my old friend.

He has become successful in many ways. He is a wonderful family man, always
concerned about his children, especially the ones who need him the most. He is charitable
with his time in helping people. He has become financially successful.

All in all from "Nuttin to Something" is an understatement.

Take it from someone who knew him "when".

Very truly yours,

Joel N. Gutterman, CPA
Partner

"When a man dies, if he can pass enthusiasm along to his children, he has left them an estate of
incalculable value."
~ Thomas Edison

Walter,

When I saw this quote in my Winning Attitude email this morning, you were the first person that came
to mind.... And, not for the dying part either! :)

I will be forever grateful to your invaluable lessons on enthusiasm; an education more valuable than
any book, lecture and class that I have ever taken.

Thank you for your priceless gift.

Happy and Healthy New Year.

Gabe

Walter: For you to share with publisher : On our journey through life we meet thousands of people and there are always a select few who make an indelible impression on us. Walter is one of those few whose sense of purpose in life is the most resolute I have ever witnessed. His love of family and friends and his fierce independence and drive are his trademarks. His urging to be the best you can be is the foundation of his being and that spirit touches everyone . For Walter adversity is a mere bump in the road on the way to the top of the mountain! It is an honor to be counted in his circle of friends. Peter

walter is a person with a great heart for helping other people when they are sick or in need. i feel it is a previlage for me and my wife to know him and his family for all these years. i wish walter nothing but health and happyness for a long and prosperous life. love and well wishes bruce and diana treitler.

Denise Brown, Disney

When I first met Walter, we had an instant connection. Although we meet at a party and only spoke for a limited time, I knew immediately that I not only liked him, but more importantly, I trusted him. Ever since then Walter has been a tremendous source of inspiration for me. He has seen me through good times and bad – and I'm grateful for both. My friendship with Walter has made the good times in my life better, and has helped me not only survive the bad times, but learn from them. In addition to being there for me, and all that I have learned from him in those times, I've also gained tremendous insight on life by observing him when he has _one through good times and bad. In the worst of times, he still sees the best there is to see – he sees the positive that most of us miss when we are down, and that some of us miss even on our best day. He has asked me many a time "How may I help you?" He has helped me in many ways, but the bottom line is that he always helps me by loving me – not just with his heart, but also with his actions -- listening, advising and spending time together.

ACKNOWLEDGEMENTS
by M. Walter Levine

There are so many people I need to offer my heartfelt thanks and appreciation. Some of you have stuck by me during my darkest hours, and I'll never forget you. Without you, it could never work for me. So thank you to my family & friends in business and in life.

In addition to my great children and my super grandchildren, I'd also like to give a shout out to my children's partners in love and life. My daughter, Leslie's, husband, Gregg Oxfeld is also a very important member of our family. He is hard working and devoted to his family, with a true gift for preparing amazing feasts. He has a degree from the Culinary Institute of America, and we've been the lucky recipients of his talent in the kitchen, many times for many years and more to come. Although Gregg travels regularly for his job with a large security company, he manages to make lots of time for the most important things in life to him — being with Leslie and his 3 children and doing charity work. He is rightfully proud of his role as parent, and he and Leslie deserve praise for the job they've done bringing up three amazing children, Sara, Andrew, and Nikki.

My daughter, Lori's husband Ray Esposito, is a very good man, a great son-in-law and the "Jack of all Trades" in our family. He's a devoted and loving husband to Lori and a wonderful father to his fantastic kids, Jamie and Julie. Ray's truly the guru of all things technical in our family. When anything is broken, not working right or just too complicated to understand, Ray can handle it, fix it, install it or replace it. His kind nature and friendly personality fits very well with Lori, and their focus on their family is a beautiful thing to see. Ray has a career that he enjoys and does very well, one of the top engineers with Stanley Black and Decker.

And of course, there's Steve's wife, Barbara, a wonderful wife and mother to their two children, Brittney and Brian, who bring me great joy and pride. Barbara and Steve have done an excellent job of building a devoted family. Our family wouldn't be the same without all of you in it, and I love you all. With my kids, we've enjoyed so many years of travel — family vacations have been (and still are) the best! The Bahamas, Disney World, Las Vegas, Puerto Rico, Mexico - tremendous laughter, joy and love shared with my loved ones.

Diana, I believe that our chance meeting was Beshert (God's will) and meant to be. They say that life is about timing, and I'll be forever grateful to Ivan who insisted that I come with him to Las Vegas (and of course, the friends and family that enabled me to go). You have come into my life for a reason and I'm very thankful for all of your love and support. Our story has turned into a love story and proves the point that no one should be alone. Love can grow and life can be wonderful together. We have spent the better part of 2 years getting to know, respect, and love each other. I look forward to sharing our lives together for the next 30 years.

Another regular fixture in my life, and indeed now a part of my family, is my right arm, KB (Kathy Beck). She is a gem and takes care of so much during my hectic workweek that it's truly amazing. She feels the needs of the patients we take care of daily. She runs to get boxes of TBL-12/Sea Cucumber for people that stop by and takes care of the bills with great care. She puts the question, "How Can I Help You?" into practice daily, with love and professionalism, and she has worked constantly and tirelessly to help make this book into a great story. It was a very lucky day in December of 2007 when KB appeared! I'm so very blessed and extremely grateful to have her as a friend and assistant. Her fiancé, Curtis, is one fortunate man to have won the heart of this kind and intelligent lady. He's been adopted to work the Pro Sports Challenge with us as well. I love working with you KB — we're a great team. Thanks for everything. I couldn't get by without you. I hope you know that.

Besides Virginia, KB and Cousin Inky, there is a special lady by the name of Linda Keppler who worked with me 30 years ago and came back into my life to help ghost write this book. She spent many hours, days and weeks, wading through all of my chicken scratch to help me craft the stories that came from my heart. She worked from her home in Reno as well as my office in CT to help put this book together. I know it would never have happened without her daily work and dedication. You, once again, have earned my respect and admiration. You are a very proud and wonderful person with a giant heart. I appreciate the daily chats while you were working day and night to get this done. I tried as hard as I could to create something that people could read and take away the thought: "If he could do it, so could I. If he could beat poor, then so could I. If he could beat cancer, and so could I!" Linda, I think we've done just that. I am forever grateful. Thank you. I hope you feel the emotion.

I'd like to give a big round of applause to my other son, Leroy Johnson and his wife, Louise, who were always around our home and business to help out when needed. Whether it was Larry's fundraiser, the Pro Sports Challenge, or just ensuring our home and businesses ran like clockwork, Leroy could always be counted on. From his early days as a supervisor with our alarm company, and all through the 28 years we've been blessed to know him, Leroy has been like a third son to me. I know Fritzie felt the same way, and the time working in her gardens with him, were some of her happiest. His assistant, JR, has also been a tremendous help throughout the years. Leroy makes things happen and always with a smile and enormous energy. His brother, Ronald, deserves mention too, another wonderful guy, always there to lend a hand. From our family to yours, your years of service and friendship are most appreciated. Thanks Lee for taking care of our patients and clients daily.

God bless you Carole and Don Sherman. How you found the time to leave your work and help pack up my entire house, and throw out almost everything I had (kidding), is something I will be eternally grateful for, I think. You helped make the transition and move work. You are my brother and sister, and I am always there for you. I am also so grateful to Marcia and Donald Siegelaub, and Mary (at 103). Thank you to Jaye and Joe Sweedler and their families for taking me in and watching over me during a very tough time in my life. I appreciate your sharing your home and dinners with me, and just for being there. I love you all.

I want to say thanks again to Gad Selig, associate Dean of Business Development University of Bridgeport and University of Bridgeport President Neil Salonen who gave me my start in the world of higher education at the University of Bridgeport with my lecture series. His son Gabe is an attorney and a really fun guy — thoughtful, smart and living the dream. I enjoy having him as a friend and neighbor. Much gratitude to the Selig men for the opportunities and warm feelings your friendship has always brought. I appreciate the introduction to intellectual higher education affairs of Bridgeport.

I've enjoyed playing craps (dice) since the excitement of the game got a hold of me in 1964 at the Flamingo Hotel in Las Vegas. Over the years, we would take all of the grandkids to Las Vegas to see shows and spend quality time together, and we enjoyed becoming friends with Charlie Meyerson from Steve Wynn's hotels. Charlie and his staff, Steve Battaglini and Michelle Rapose, took very special care of everything and were absolutely wonderful to our family. Thanks to Steve Wynn and the Wynn Hotel and the Encore. I still visit as often as possible. You are my family on the West Coast.

One time High Speed Video had a booth at the Las Vegas Convention Center and we found out that we had to rent a TV for $800 a day from the Convention Center to show our production. I thought that was a waste of money and thought it would be better to buy a television, use it for the four days of the convention, then donate it. So I called Steve Wynn and asked if he knew of a charity in Las Vegas for children that I could donate it to. He directed me to his wife, Elaine. Working together, HSV bought a 60" screen TV that we used for the four days, and we were able to donate the $1,200 television to the Wynn's Children's Charity. It was a Wynn/Wynn situation! Yes, it can be done!

There are so very many special residents of Little Rock who will hold a place in my heart forever. As I've said, they are like family to me. I still cherish my time with them when I went for my check-ups. One angel in particular is Bonnie Jenkins at the Arkansas Cancer Research Center. Sonia, you're amazing behind the scenes – simply terrific. To Stephanie

Simington, who helped me think of the future as worthy of the vision. And to all the other special people in Arkansas, thanks again. You are my Arkansas family.

Thanks to Dr. Sundar Jagannath and Stephanie Stoss, and all the impressive folks at St Vincent's Comprehensive Cancer Center (which has since moved to Mt. Sinai) in NYC, where the trials on the TBL-12 Sea Cucumber products are being done. The same ones that I take every day to help, I believe, cure my cancer. The patients whom I refer to Dr. Jagannath in NYC are grateful. The staff is amazing — they truly care, and it's not about the money. It comes from their heart, and you can feel it. There are some very special doctors and nurses in so many hospitals around the world. You're very lucky if you are working with a hospital of your choice, one that makes a difference. I hope you get that lucky.

A huge amount of gratitude goes to Herb and Helen Gordon for bringing TBL-12/Sea Cucumber home from Australia for me and for introducing me to Sam Grant. What can I say? You guys changed my life, and I'm thrilled to be Sam's U.S. Distributor, working as a not-for-profit. I am privileged and determined to ensure that we continue to help people get the TBL-12 Dietary Food Supplement product, and I thank God that I've been able to get the product to as many people as I have. There's been a great success rate and I look forward to the day the medical trials conclude and there is official approval by the medical profession and the FDA.

I want to say a big thank you to Fed Ex. If these good guys didn't deliver the very next morning, we would have no chance of saving the amount of lives that we do with TBL-12. They take the product and help to keep it frozen and deliver it to our patients in the perfect condition, so they can continue to take it and try to stay healthy. Thank you Lenny, Lou and Nick Esposito for coming up with the pure genius of another entrepreneurial idea that worked.

Another special person is David Fishof, an agent for sports and entertainment personalities such as Ringo Starr, football players like Phil

Simms, as well as other celebs. As I was dealing with the cancer treatments, David would often call to have me join him for lunch, dinner or a Broadway show. The outpouring of support and friendship from him and so many others gave me an even stronger fighting spirit to beat the cancer. I knew that I had to take this massive show of kindness and affection, to pay it forward, and to pass the good vibes on. I wanted to share the feelings of hope and inspiration that I was so lucky to receive from so many.

A special thanks to John Capozzi, who has been an inspiration and true advisor throughout this book writing, production, marketing and publishing process. Your expertise has served me well.

You just have to look at the possibilities of life. We are all responsible for our own futures. No matter how difficult the times are, it's up to us to survive, thrive and love. It's all about the heart of a person, the heart of the people and spirituality in a world of uncertainty. The best is yet to come. Think positive! I've said it before and I'll say it again, if you don't ask and shoot for the moon and stars, it's akin to winking at a girl in the dark — you know what you're doing, but nobody else does. So ask, and never stop asking. Dreams are wonderful things. They are how things get done. A wish is a dream your heart makes. You've got to dream it, visualize it and then do it. I learned that if you are going to make it in life, no matter what you do, you have an obligation to yourself and others to do it to the very best of your ability. Have a plan of how you would like to see it, and see things through to the point that you get personal satisfaction. Win, lose or draw, at least you know you gave it your best shot with passion. If it doesn't work out, you can always try again, and you'll try even harder next time.

I promised to finish this book, which I began almost twelve years ago, as a story to share with my family. It has grown into a desire to help as many people as I can believe that the fight to live never ends. Don't let it end — the more you believe, the more you can conceive. During my illness, people seemed to come from out of the woodwork to give me such an abundance of love and support. I felt so very blessed, and I truly don't think I'll ever be able to communicate just how much their show of love meant to me. To me, relationships are everything. Relationships mean that you need each other. I wish I could put it on the bottom of each page of this book: Build Relationships! Relationships build you! Friends, family and business — that's what keeps me going. Have I mentioned what a lucky guy I am? Thank you to all of you who make my life blessed. What would I do without you?

My life is filled with special people and relationships that could fill the pages of hundreds of books, so it's impossible to list them all and give them all the proper due. But please know that each member of my family and my "family of friends" are the most important part of my life. The 200+ calls I get and make during the week and another 100 on the weekends warms my heart. So thank you for being in my life. To have a friend, you have to be a friend, and, boy....do I have friends! One and all, I love you all!

www.mwalterlevine.com

ACKNOWLEDGEMENTS
by Virginia Juliano

Although this is Walter's book, not mine, it did take a lot of time, effort and sacrifice on my part to get it to where it is, and I want to thank several people for helping me get it, and me, to the finish line:

First and foremost, my husband, Charles Gasperino (aka Gasparino), who has always been my biggest fan and supporter. Chuck, you always pushed me to see what was possible and to think "beyond," despite how silly or unrealistic it might seem to others. Thanks for pulling me through during my meltdowns when I thought I could not write another word. To my Mom, Angela Garone Juliano, who has always wanted the best for me and loved me even when I was a bratty, depressive teenager. I love to watch you become a kid again with your grandchildren. It's a beautiful thing to see.

My sister, Tina Juliano DiSalvo, who understands me without words. I'm continuously impressed at what a wonderful woman and mother you've grown up to be. Her husband Joseph DiSalvo, who I've known since he was a kid. Joe you are my little brother and couldn't imagine our family without you. Matthew and Mia, my darling nephew and niece, whom I adore. Sorry that I have to smother you both with kisses every time I see you, but you're so cute, I just can't help myself. To my father Raffaele Iuliano, who despite our differences, I've learned a great deal from. James Gasparino, my brother in law. I'm so happy to have you as part of our family, and always appreciate being able to create family memories with you (and of course, the free, and always spot-on, medical advice). My late grandfather, Philip Garone, who taught me to be self-sufficient, independent and an original thinker. You were the best, and I still miss you every day.

Aunt Phyllis and Uncle Benny Giannone, who are my Godparents and have always been there for me. Thank you for everything. My cousins, Peter and Nicole, and Michael and Lauren Giannone — I can't imagine the holidays without you. I wish our lives weren't so hectic and we'd be able to see each other more than once a year. Aunt Roseanne, Uncle Robert and Steven Bergman. Much love and kisses.

My oldest and dearest friend, Sandy Cangiano Noll. I'm so glad you asked me what my name was that fateful day in the schoolyard of P.S. 132. Even when we don't talk for months, as soon as we do, we're exactly back to where we left off. That's a best friend. My dear Denis Gawley, who never fails to crack me up. You are a sweet man and it's such a blessing to have you in my life. My girls, Catherine Tracey and Andrea Parsons. Many years of laughter and tears have made us much more than friends. We are truly soul sisters and I can't imagine my life in New York without you both. Sheryl (Serena) Hankins, I miss you, and hope you are at peace. Linda F., you rock, and I'm so glad that we've become friends. It feels like we've known each other forever.

My former co-workers at M. Shanken Communications, Inc., where I started my career and basically grew up. We had some fun, fun times. My colleagues at Showtime Networks Inc. – I couldn't ask for a more professional, interesting and plain old nice group of people to work with. Thanks to Ann and the group for keeping me honest. And of course, to Walter, who changed my life one August day in Westport. Thanks for seeing something in me that I didn't even see in myself.